A Life of Natural Health

by Merrilyn Hope

A Life of Natural Health

Disclaimer

This book is designed as a guide only, not as a medical manual. The ideas herein are only suggestions to help you make informed choices about your health and the health of your family. The ideas expressed are not intended as a replacement for any medication or therapy you have been prescribed by your doctor or alternative health practitioner. The author takes no responsibility for the effects of any treatment or remedy which you may try. Please make sure to discuss your health options with your doctor or health professional before trying out any of these cleansing processes, diets, herbs, vitamins, exercises, meditation and breathing techniques, homeopathic remedies, or anything else suggested herein.

Contents

Forward

I have practiced natural methods of healing for at least forty years, however, in my early life I gained qualifications in music, with an LTCL for piano and an A.Mus. in music theory (and more recently, a B.A. in art history). I currently teach both music and yoga and promote awareness of alternative therapies on my website, www.merrilynhope.com.

In 1984 I self-published my first health book, entitled 'No Cancer Notebook'. This was followed by 'The No Cancer And Candida Notebook' in 1990, which was published by an Auckland publisher and distributor. In these books, I stressed the importance of a wheat free and dairy free diet in healing the illnesses we had experienced as a result of poisonous herbicide exposure. At the time, these ideas were regarded as 'wayout' by many people. Nowadays, over thirty years later, some of my previous critics are proponents of either the 'gluten free' diet, which achieves more or less the same result as the old 'wheat free' one, or they follow a dairy free diet and use soya milk instead of cow's milk.

My interest became a serious study after the births of my children, when I observed the effects of certain vaccinations and toxic herbicides on their health. My firstborn child had just two vaccinations which made him severely ill, after which I endeavoured to not vaccinate ever again, and instead, to use homeopathic and natural methods as alternatives to conventional medicine.

Since writing my health books, which were done for the purpose of helping people with the marvellous diets and healing techniques I had discovered, my sons set up a health and environment website for me to write on.

The MerrilynHope.com website, which has been running for nearly ten years now, has proved a successful platform to bring many health and environmental issues to light.

My sons and my daughter have been urging me to 'do' another book for quite a while. I am grateful for their valuable advice and their technical and creative input.

Many thanks to Lachlan MacKinven for getting me started on this project, and for producing this book so stylishly.

Thank you especially to Holly MacKinven for her lovely, eye-catching cover design.

Thank you to Mathilde Cruchet for the beautiful book layout.

I also acknowledge my other two sons, Alexis Hope, who published the E book version for me on Amazon, and Isadore William Crooks, and give acknowledgment to healers Walter Last, and Bernhard Petersen. They have all had a major influence on my life and on my thinking.

Thanks also to Dr. Max Gerson and the many healers whose books I have read and learnt from. Hopefully, this collection of the most relevant articles from the website, which have been expanded in most cases, will provide food for thought for all those people who are interested in preventing disease and keeping good health.

NOTE: Although I would take the alternative approach every time, readers should not necessarily follow my advice. Different things work for different people. DO see a doctor or a suitably qualified health professional if you are sick, or you think you may have cancer or some other degenerative disease.

Chapter 1

Nutritional Deficiencies, Toxic Chemicals And Their Effect On Health

'We are a health system that keeps sick people alive and we do very little in reversing the problem.' (Professor Ian Brighthope).

Mineral-deficient soils, combined with the use of superphosphate fertiliser and other toxic agrichemicals, could be the real causes of cancer and other degenerative disease. Foods grown on depleted soils, and the animals which graze on them, are deficient in the important, sustaining elements of life. This problem is compounded when toxic herbicides and pesticides are used in our environment and on the food which we eat.

I have had my own unfortunate experiences with poisonous agrichemicals such as 2,4,5-T, (called 'Agent Orange' in VietNam), Dieldrin, RoundUp and various others.
But these are the very experiences which have heightened my awareness and sensitivity as to the harmful effects of agricultural poisons, and which have prompted me to write about them in the hope that people may protect their health better and avoid devastating illnesses.
Many of my more cynical friends, who rejected naturopathic methods for treating disease, and who regularly used herbicides and pesticides, have gone to early graves after the failure of conventional treatments for their cancers and heart disease.
I can identify the exposure to certain chemicals as being the cause of chronic ill health at various times in my life – I am certain that aerial spraying with

2,4,5-T, which was sprayed directly over our rural house, and which poisoned our water supply, was the cause of years of ill health for my young son and myself, and contributed to the death of our baby daughter.

The other poisoning factor in our lives around this time was the drinking of milk from cows fed on pastures which were being regularly sprayed:

Although our milk was unpasteurised, and very fresh, it was still very bad for the health, as it contained all the poisons being used on the paddocks, such as glyphosate, 2,4,5-T and superphosphate.

Although dairy boards monitor the milk and declare a certain amount of herbicide and pesticide to be 'safe', their assurances should be taken with a grain of salt, as there is no such thing as as a safe amount of poison. Some people are more vulnerable than others.

The later essay in this book on 'Bee Colony Collapse Disorder' will tell you why even such small amounts of poison, as to be undetectable by modern technology, can have such a disastrous effect on small insects such as bees. We could assume from the research done on bees, that humans could be being similarly affected by miniscule amounts of poisons such as glyphosate and other herbicides and pesticides. Even antibiotics themselves are affected by herbicides such as glyphosate. See http://merrilynhope.com/antibiotic-medicine-harmed-by-herbicides-including-roundup/

Following the advice of Walter Last (natural therapist and author) on our very serious illness after the 2,4,5-T spraying, we began a cleansing regime, and adopted a predominantly raw-food diet. No dairy milk, sugar or wheat was allowed. This was the only way to what was to be a very slow but sure recovery.

Such is my personal experience of the effects of hormone sprays such as 2,4,5-T, and 2,4-D. These chemicals were used during the Vietnam war with dreadful consequences and, thankfully, they have since been banned.

Now we need to beware of the other poisonous chemicals which have taken their place, such as glyphosate, which is found in the common weed-killer, RoundUp, and 1080, brodifacoum, neonic-otinoids, and many other herbicides and pesticides which also have the potential to kill birds, bees and harm humans and animals alike.

Glyphosate-containing RoundUp, I find, is very harmful to the health, as it readily kills off the beneficial organisms in the bowel, and causes the harmful ones to proliferate. This can set the stage for cancer and arthritis to develop, as well as nervous ailments. For many years glyphosate has been insistently marketed as a 'safe' product, despite the bad reactions many of us have to it. This status is changing. The World Health Organisation recently, in March, 2015, declared that glyphosate 'probably' causes cancer. The fear of being sued by the companies who manufacture the weedkiller is probably the reason for their seemingly indecisive statement, which is conveniently diluted to placate the big chemical giants, in my opinion.

The following excerpt is quoted from Andrew Porterfield, July 24th, 2015, 'Genetic Literacy Project'. (geneticliteracyproject.org)

'In March, the World Health Organisation's International Agency for Research on Cancer, IARC,
issued a statement (also published in The Lancet) that reclassified glyphosate as 'probably carcinogenic to humans'. It was a surprise to some in the scientific community because every major regulatory agency had determined that glyphosate, an herbicide often paired with genetically modified crops, was not carcinogenic.'

The Trouble With Superphosphate

Superphosphate, an agricultural fertiliser, is another damaging product widely used in commercial farming practice. Like glyphosate in RoundUp, it is difficult to avoid. In farming communities it is in the air we breathe, gets into our rivers and our water supply, and most foods we buy are contaminated with it.

Superphosphate fertiliser is causing on-going problems with people's health today. Percy Weston's account of his careful farming and animal studies, which were undertaken over many years, suggest that the artificial fertiliser superphosphate is contributing to the epidemics of cancer, arthritis, parkinson's disease, and many other health problems in society today. See the book by Percy Weston:

'Cancer: Cause and Cure: A 20th Century Perspective' (published by Book bin, Adelaide, South Australia, 2000, 2003).

When combined with a low iodine intake, excessive phosphorus in the body can cause growths in the throat and thyroid glands, but this is only one of many diseases which can result from the prevalence of artificial phosphate in our food.

Artificial superphosphate contains other contaminants besides phosphorus: Traces of cadmium, which is extremely hazardous to health, is found in artificial fertiliser. Cadmium, combined with phosphorus, is one main cause of heart disease becoming so prevalent in Australia, according to Percy Weston. Weston also observed that high phosphate levels were to blame in sudden cases of polio with family members, and warns about artificial superphosphate as being a probable contributor in cot deaths, child asthma, and other child maladies. This is one major reason for avoiding standard, pasteurised dairy milk. Weston insists that raw milk from organically treated pastures should be the only milk taken in treating disease, and in preserving health.

For many years I have suspected that superphosphate fertiliser was bad for the health: I always had an extreme reaction to it whenever I visited one particular family who used it on their dairy farm. Even if the paddocks were not being treated, the house and furniture always smelled strongly of superphosphate. One member of this family had chronic asthma over all the years he lived on the farm. I was certain superphosphate was the main protagonist in his bouts of asthma, as I had asthma-type symptoms whenever I stayed there.

Two other members of this family suffer high blood pressure and heart problems. I believe these can be attributed to superphosphate and cadmium, as well as the use of RoundUp. The glyphosate-containing RoundUp came next on the list of allergy-causing agrichemicals which were used on their farm. Both superphosphate and RoundUp are currently still widely used on virtually every non-organic farm in New Zealand. And, alarmingly, glyphosate-containing RoundUp is considered safe by many organic farmers and orchardists in New Zealand who use it when, quite clearly, it is not safe.

The 'RoundUp', glyphosate weedkiller has been sold to the world for decades under the pretence that it was 'biodegradable'. It was only about two years ago that the manufacturers were forced to remove the 'biodegradable' claim from their advertising.

My belief is that glyphosate has no place on any organic farm, and farms which use it should not be allowed to label their food as organic.

Phosphorus Linked To Parasites And Cancer

Phosphorus is difficult to eliminate without the help of a low-phosphorus diet, which includes raw vegetables, fruit, and juices. Left unchecked, excess phosphorus will encourage pathogens and parasites to develop in the digestive tract and intestines. These can escape into the bloodstream and end up in the liver, kidneys, and other organs. Percy Weston is convinced, as are many naturopaths and doctors such as Walter Last, and Dr. Hulda Regehr Clark, that there is a direct relationship between parasites and cancer.

Methods For Eradicating Harmful Parasites

Walter Last's theory was that dairy products themselves, especially pasteurised milk, and wheat, were the main cause of intestinal parasites. Milk causes mucous, which harbours intestinal worms of many descriptions. He believed that a milk-free, wheat-free, sugar-free diet was best in curing disease, and that without milk, cheese, wheat or sugar in the diet, intestinal parasites would not survive.
Walter advised eating garlic with every meal to avoid infestation of parasites.
Fasting for several days on unsweetened lemon drink, or eating only grated raw apple, or grated carrot, will remove intestinal parasites.

Dr. Clark maintains, as does Walter Last, that killing intestinal parasites is imperative in curing cancer. She uses a traditional recipe which includes black walnut hulls. This, she says, will kill all parasites within a week. See Chapter 5, 'Cancer Doctor's Treatment Uses Just Three Herbs' for details on the traditional black walnut, artemisia and cloves recipe for getting rid of intestinal parasites and curing cancer.

How Arthritis And Cancer Were Healed With Epsom Salts

Shortly after being exposed to hormone sprays, Percy Weston developed an extremely pernicious cancer which was growing rapidly along the back of his hand. He was advised by a doctor to have radium treatment, but since his own doctor of many years, as well as another friend, had both just died of cancer after unsuccessful radium treatments, he decided to devise his own therapy.

Weston decided on Epsom Salts, which is magnesium sulphate. This alone is a remedy for constipation and will remove toxins and parasites from the digestive system. It also neutralises acid in the body. He mixed Epsom Salts with bicarbonate of soda and sulphates of potassium and iron. His self-prescribed dose was initially a quarter teaspoon per day, taken in lemon juice. This dose of salts was built up to a teaspoonful per day.

The Epsom Salt combination was an incredible success. His long-standing arthritis began immediately to improve, and after a month, the cancer became smaller, with new, healthy growth gradually replacing the cancer. Within six months, both arthritis and cancer had disappeared, and except for a slight recurrence of arthritis in one knee, these illnesses never bothered him again.

The Importance Of Bowel Cleansing

Sulphur is a strong antiseptic, and also keeps the bowels clean. Intestinal parasites do not like Sulphur, so a dose of Sulphur can eradicate worms such as fluke in animals, as well as humans.

Lice and other parasites are attracted to animals which are deficient in Sulphur. The appearance of lice is usually an indication that the animal, or human, is minerally deficient, and not in optimum health. Percy Weston used an application of powdered Sulphur along the spine of affected cattle, which removed lice within about five hours or so.

Our forebears were in the habit of clearing the intestines with either a weekly dose of castor oil, or Epsom Salts, or a mixture of sulphur and treacle. Our health would be all the better for taking up this practice again, as it would regularly remove cancer-causing parasites from the bowel and get rid of effete matter. See later chapters in this book on the use of castor oil in treating cancer and arthritis.

Note: The homeopathic remedy Sulphur is often recommended to remove intestinal worms, but this treatment needs to be combined with an appropriate diet: as Walter Last believed, it is best to remove milk from the diet when worms are persistent. Intestinal parasites thrive on milk, and their prevalence can lead to cancer, as they produce harmful toxins which are absorbed into the blood. It is important to get rid of them.

The Benefits Of Letting A Cold Run Its Course

Getting a cold or the flu gives the body a chance to expel excess phosphorus from the blood, as well as numerous other unwanted toxins. It is a build-up of phosphorus and other toxins which lead to cancer and arthritis, according to Percy Weston. He states that it is no good to suppress a cold or the flu by taking aspirin or some other medication, as no toxins or phosphorus are expelled if you do that. I agree with his method entirely, although I do swear by homeopathic Arsen alb., both as a treatment and a prophylactic for flu and colds, with hot lemon drinks taken every hour. A chapter on the uses of homeopathic Arsen alb. is included later in this book.

Chapter 2

The Gerson Cancer Diet And An Example Of A Cancer Programme

Healing With Raw Foods And Castor Oil

Dr. Gerson is one of the most influential healers in the field of alternative medicine in the past fifty years. His ideas, I believe, have influenced many healers such as Walter Last, Dr. Ann Wigmore, and writers Jaquie Davison and Edie May who have written about their recoveries using his methods.

Dr. Ann Wigmore had virulent cancer which she healed with an adaptation of Dr. Gerson's methods. Her recovery was a lengthy process, partly due to the disbelief of the medical profession. Her medical peers insisted on her having a biopsy after six months of her alternative treatment, as they did not believe she could have had cancer. Cancer, they said, could not be cured through following a specific diet. The biopsy procedure, which certainly did prove she had cancer, caused the cancer to reactivate itself. She went back onto her healing diet and cleansing. This time, it took two years of treatment to recover properly. After healing herself of the dreaded disease, she started healing clinics of her own. Many people attending her clinics, one of which was in Sydney, Australia, have recovered from cancer and other degenerative diseases using her alternative treatments. In essence, Dr. Gerson did not believe in chemotherapy or radiation treatment. He believed that cancer, which develops over time in a toxic, acid body, can be reversed when potassium-rich vegetables and fruits replace the acid-forming foods, and detoxification methods are used.

Castor oil and enemas are an integral part of his treatments. Castor oil is a great healer, and has the ability to draw toxins from the organs, tissues and blood. The enemas are also vital to a quick recovery, as they wash away the toxins quickly which are being released from the liver due to the cleansing raw foods and castor oil. Without enemas, these poisons

which are expelled into the intestines, travel slowly enough to be absorbed back into the blood through the walls of the bowel.
Enemas prevent the reabsorption of toxins through the bowel walls.
Jaquie Davison grew new tooth enamel, and a new head of healthy hair after a year of following Gerson's castor oil and juice regime to cure her melanoma. She began the treatment after being told by her doctor that she had just three weeks to live. She was bedridden at the time.
See Jaquie Davison's book, 'Cancer Winner: How I Purged Myself of Melanoma', 1977.
Thanks to the persistence of her daughter, who had read about the Gerson diet, the prediction of the doctors did not prove correct: she recovered completely, and went on to write a book about her miraculous recovery.
I am confident that Dr. Gerson's healing methods work. In fact, I have healed myself using his methods, first when I had a breast lump, and then later at various times when environmental pollution had got the better of me.

In a nutshell, here is an adapted version of the Gerson diet which I used to eliminate the lump in my breast:
1) A bowl of oatmeal porridge every morning, taken with a grated, raw apple which has its skin left on. No sugar or dairy milk is taken with the porridge. Walter Last allowed a little butter, but no other dairy products. However, in the early days of treating cancer, it is probably better to do without the butter.
No other cooked food in the diet initially, except for the morning porridge.
2) Castor oil every second day at 10 o'clock. The dose is 2 tablespoons.
This is followed by an enema within five hours af-

ter the castor oil. Take more enemas throughout the day, whenever nausea is felt. Make sure to have at least three enemas per day.

3) Vegetable and fruit juices taken by the glassful every hour.
Salads of fresh, raw vegetables for lunch and tea.
No bread, or dairy foods except for butter, no sugar, no wheat, no cooked foods: all foods are eaten raw.

4) Liver juice for enzymes is taken in sips through-out the day. Both Dr. Gerson and Walter Last used this in their treatments for cancer and other degenerative conditions.

Example Of My Dietary Programme For The Day

This illustrates how I spent a typical day when treating the lump in my breast many years ago. It is an adaptation of the approaches of Dr. Gerson and Walter Last. It worked. After three months, the lump had gone. It began to grow again when I gave up the diet, but after resuming the diet with castor oil and enemas, it eventually disappeared for good.

I sent the following programme to a friend of mine who had only three weeks to live. This article originally appeared on my website blog, entitled: Cancer Programme For Anthony. I have not heard from him since, so it is possible that he did not attempt the diet and has passed away. He lived in Wellington, New Zealand, and I had moved North to Auckland, so I had already lost touch with him.

Diet, Castor Oil, And Enemas: A Letter To A Friend

Hello Anthony, I haven't heard how you are getting along. I hope you are managing to keep positive about life and that you have started the programme.

There really is nothing to lose by giving it your best shot if allopathic medicine cannot help you any longer.

If you have had chemotherapy and radiation, then your immune system will be weakened considerably. This makes it harder to recover on a mainly raw foods and enema/castor oil programme, but some people have achieved this despite having had chemotherapy and radiation. Recovery IS still possible.

Determination is the key. An understanding of how the treatment works is also necessary, because then you will put all your effort into doing the things that will make you well: detoxifying the body quickly is imperative if you are to beat the growth of the cancer and assist the immune system into doing its work effectively again.

Leaving out some things completely also assists the immune system: all coffee, tea, alcohol, dairy products, wheat, cooked food except for morning porridge, must be omitted for the duration of your recovery (except for the coffee taken with castor oil, and possibly coffee enemas).

There are three main constituents of the programme which serve to help the body detoxify quickly: Diet, Castor Oil, and Enemas. I have included Vitamin C as the fourth detoxifier, with Breathing and Exercise as the fifth detoxifiers:

1. Diet

Eat mainly raw foods, with a large plate of oatmeal porridge every morning, eaten with a grated apple. The bulk of raw foods, and the porridge also, helps to clean out the digestive system including the bowel. The intestines are where most problems start for people, as old undigested food sits around in pockets where putrefying organisms breed. Toxins from eating mucous forming foods (such as milk and cheese, wheat bread, to name a few) which are not digested or eliminated properly from the bowel, can lead to cancer cells proliferating.

Often our diets do not include enough raw food in proportion to the cooked foods we are eating. Roughage in the form of raw foods is important in treating cancerous conditions and other degenerative disease. Also, once the bowel is clean and more raw foods, and later, cooked vegetables, are included in the diet, the digestion improves as your intestines become capable of absorbing more of the nutrients from the food you eat.

The diet for treating degenerative disease is a maintenance diet which is easily digested and cleansing: juices and raw foods provide optimum nutrition which aid the immune system and healing; at the same time, a drastic reduction in acid-forming foods, cooked food and mucous-forming foods helps prevent the cancer from growing.

Note: Almonds and two raw egg yolks per day can be included in the diet after an initial period of cleansing, which should take about three weeks.

Use plenty of garlic right from the beginning of the treatment: try to have some with your salads or right after each meal.

Apricot kernels, or peach or nectarine kernels, contain laetrile and organic cyanide which have been found to be helpful in treating cancer and reducing growths. Read Cancer Research UK, cancerresearchuk.org ,for more information on laetrile, also known as vitamin B17 or amygdalin.

Almonds and peach kernels contain small amounts of laetrile and cyanide, but apricot kernels have higher levels. I used organic apricot kernels in my treatment of a breast lump. Following the guidelines I have given in this post to you, it took three months for the lump to reduce dramatically, then another three months before it disappeared forever.

I began with about three or four apricot kernels a day, and gradually increased the amount to nine per day, which were taken two or three at a time after my salad meals. If you include apricot kernels in your diet, then it is imperative that you follow through with the enema treatment, otherwise too much cyanide will remain in the intestines. Nine kernels a day should be a safe amount, considering that regular enemas will eliminate the excess cyanide from the system, but do get some advice as to the amount which is suitable for you. Body weight has a bearing on how many you should have.

2. Castor Oil

This is a great detoxifier which is helpful in cancerous conditions. Castor oil has powerful healing properties. It also has the ability to attract poisons, and most importantly, poisons from the liver and bowel, which are then easily eliminated via the castor oil from the body.

3. Enemas

See the Chapter 32 'How Enemas Can Help Cancer And Arthritis' for more information on the use of enemas for healing degenerative disease.
These are very important. The more severe your sickness, the more developed the cancer, then the more urgency there is to begin enema treatment to speed up the detoxification process.

4. Vitamins

Some healers, like Walter Last, believe that extra vitamins are not necessary if you are on a diet which is 90% raw food obtained from organic sources: Eat fresh fruit and vegetables and drink their juices often throughout the day.
However, I have found Calcium Ascorbate, Vitamin C powder, which is a non-acidic form of vitamin C, to be very helpful in reducing toxins from the body and in aiding healing. Vitamin C in large doses has

been found to reduce the pain of cancer, as well as to inhibit the growth of cancers, which is another good reason to invest in a quality non-acidic form of Vitamin C such as calcium ascorbate.

1000 mg morning and night is a minimum dose for a life-threatening disease. You could take up to 10,000 mg daily. Every second morning, on the day when you take your castor oil, you should take the Calcium Ascorbate powder or tablets first thing in the morning, or at lunch time, two hours before or after the dose of castor oil. This is so that the effect of the Vitamin C will not be negated by taking the Vitamin C too close to the castor oil.

5. Breathing, Meditation, Exercise

These all help one way or another to relieve stress, help create peace within the mind, and to oxygenate the body. Best of all, do the 'Exercise for Increasing Prana' breathing exercise three times a day. Do 'Yoga Nidra' deep relaxation, or the 'Yoga of Sleep' every day, preferably after lunch. (See the end chapters in this book for instructions on how to do this).

A Note On Radiation And Electrical Interference

While you are recovering, try to avoid exposure to high tension wires, cell phone towers, big transformers at the front of houses, and 'smart' meters. Make sure you are sleeping at least twelve feet away from the electricity meter box in the house where you are living. Increase the distance for a 'smart' meter, which now emits excessive amounts of radiation from microwaves.

Try to ascertain where the main power supply runs into the house and towards the meter box, and keep clear of this. Electrical interference can undermine one's health rapidly and interfere with healing. Limit the use of your cell phone, and keep it in another room from where you sleep. If you are doing your meditation or Yoga Nidra, then put the phone elsewhere. Avoid carrying it around with you.

P.S. Hi again Anthony. By now you will be going well with your cleansing programme and are hopefully into your second week or so. You could introduce the calf liver broth at this stage. Sip the juice throughout the day. I have just put up a post on calf liver juice for cancer which gives the details on how it is made. All the best.

Merrilyn, October 25th, 2011.

Chapter 3

Benefits Of Castor Oil In Treating Disease

The benefits of castor oil have been known for literally thousands of years.

Ricinus communis is the botanical name of the castor oil plant. It is sometimes referred to as the Palma Christi, the Palm of Christ, in old herbals. The 16th century herbalist John Gerard refers to the plant by this name. The more contemporary herbalist John Lust discusses the attributes of the castor oil plant and lists Palma Christi as one of its common names. The Palma Christi, or castor oil plant does have incredible healing properties, which is why it has been equated with the name of Christ.

The Many Uses Of Castor Oil

Castor oil is derived from the seeds of the castor oil plant. These seeds are extremely poisonous, so never try making your own castor oil remedy. Use only commercially produced castor oil, which is safe. When the oil is extracted from the seed, it leaves behind all the harmful poisons, and only retains those compounds which benefit our health.

Castor oil is most famously used as a purgative, to treat constipation and poisoning of various kinds. But it also has been used as a healing salve for centuries.

We were often given castor oil as children, on a weekly basis. I think it is a pity that this practice has fallen into decline, as taking castor oil on a weekly basis not only cleans out the bowels, but removes intestinal parasites, removes candida, and removes toxins from the liver. Having a clean liver protects one from getting cancer and other degenerative disease.

It is my opinion that Castor oil is a great cancer preventative. Dr. Gerson's cancer clinic still uses castor oil as part of the treatment in cancer recovery. The dose is two tablespoons every second day, followed by a series of enemas. The bulk of the diet is raw juices and raw foods, with the exception of a large bowl of porridge each morning, which is eaten with a grated raw apple. No dairy milk or sugar is added to the porridge. Walter Last recommended butter as an addition, but no other dairy products.

It is my belief that far less children in our polluted Western society would succumb to cancer and obesity if they were given a dose of castor oil on a weekly basis. The more toxic our environment becomes, the more necessity there is to detoxify the liver and the body generally.

Castor oil has the ability to attract poisons and hold them within the oil, which makes it a valuable medicine for treating cancer as well as cleansing the bowels and treating some cases of poisoning.

Castor oil feeds the nerves and nourishes the whole body. Taking castor oil internally helps hair growth, gives your skin a satiny smooth feel, improves the brain function, improves eyesight and does a host of other beneficial things.

This is partly because it reduces the toxins in the bowel. A clean bowel means that your bowel can function optimally, without the hindrance of toxins to spoil the absorption of vitamins. You get more goodness out of your food when your bowel is clean, and so you don't need those vitamin supplements so badly.

These benefits to the health, which castor oil bring, are also because castor oil enables the liver to perform optimally. The liver functions well when it is not overloaded with poisons, and castor oil will clear out the poisons.

The other thing about castor oil is that it contains some compounds which benefit the body's immune system and which help prevent disease: these compounds have been isolated by modern research scientists.

Castor Oil Remedy For Babies Suffering Constipation

Babies who are breastfed should not get constipation, we are told. But now and then, it does happen. Sometimes a crying baby can mean that the baby has become constipated. (Check with your doctor if your baby won't stop crying, in case there is an ear infection, or some other malady.)

Vasant Lad, in his book 'Ayurvedic Home Remedies' suggests that, for constipation in her baby, the mother smear her nipples with a little castor oil before feeding. This is just enough, in most cases, to be effective. This is such a simple remedy which will do no harm to your baby.

Chapter 4

How To Use The Castor Oil Pack

The Castor Oil Pack For Healing

The castor oil pack, as discussed earlier, is a valuable healing medium which was highly recommended by Dr. Max Gerson. Edgar Cayce, the American psychic healer, is another healer who believed in the miraculous abilities of the 'palma christi' to heal sicknesses of many kinds..

He prescribed this to many who came to see him for psychic readings regarding their health. Go to the website www.edgarcayce.org for more detail on the Edgar Cayce readings.

In New Zealand, the well-known Austrian healer, Walter Last, helped many people recover from cancer and other diseases with the help of castor oil and castor oil packs.

Castor oil packs help to remove toxins from the body. The action of the castor oil penetrates through the skin and into the body organs. It has the effect of increasing qi, or energy, and releasing pent-up energy and negative elements from the tissues.

The castor oil pack not only helps to remove toxins from the body tissues, it helps remove mucous and other matter from the intestines. It aids nutrition because it assists in the assimilation of vitamins and minerals in the digestive tract. It also helps to heal internal disturbances and helps to counteract the effects of radiation.

How To Make A Castor Oil Pack

The two essential components are castor oil and a piece of flannel, however there are a number of other points to take into consideration when making a castor oil pack. The method is outlined below.

Castor oil: a 50ml bottle will be enough.

A piece of flannel or white linen. For general use on the stomach area, you will need a piece of flannel about the size of a computer keyboard. This will be folded in half so that you end up with a thicker, squarish pad.

Note: Do not use any coloured cotton, linen, or flannel, and do not use any synthetic material. The cloth must be pure unbleached cotton, linen or wool. This is because castor oil is such a potent detoxifier, that it will react with the chemical dyes and synthetic fiber chemicals: it will draw these out, instead of acting on the poisons in your body. This will negate the healing effect, so please don't do it.

You also need a tin or a jar with a lid to be used for storing the castor oil pack in.

You will also need a piece of plastic to cover the pack with, and an old towel to go over that.

Simply pour over a cup of castor oil onto the pad. You might need more or less, depending on the size and thickness of the cloth you have selected. Cover the whole of the cloth and let the material soak up the castor oil.

Using The Castor Oil Pack

Warm up the pack gently in the tin or jar by putting this into a warm oven for about five minutes. Do not microwave, as this energy remains within the microwaved article, which will be harmful to your vital energies. Microwaving will also destroy some of the valuable properties of the castor oil. Castor oil is very sensitive to microwave radiations. Take care not to burn the castor oil, or to cook it. It should not be so hot that you cannot touch it comfortably with your bare hands when you take the container from the oven, just warm.

Alternatively, you can use the pack cold, with a covering of plastic and then an old towel, and use a hot water bottle (which is not too hot) on top of that. This works just as well, however, putting the cold pack straight onto the stomach can be uncomfort able to begin with.

Place the pack over the stomach area, or over the area which needs treatment. You can fold the cloth down for a better fit if necessary. Be generous with the size: it is good to treat as much of the stomach as you can, covering the liver area and the entire lower stomach area. This will benefit the liver, kidneys, bladder, reproductive parts, and the intestines. Place the plastic over the pack, then wrap the towel around.

The castor oil pack works best if you leave it on for at least three hours at a time, but overnight is best.

The Three Day Treatment

If you have cancer, or some other serious internal disease such as a nervous condition, then you should endeavor to keep the castor oil pack on the stomach overnight, and repeat the treatment for three days in a row. Then leave off the pack for three consecutive days before beginning the three-day treatment again. You can continue ad infinitum with this routine of three days on, three days off, until the disease has improved and your digestive function is restored. I recommend keeping a good-sized castor oil pack specifically for the treatment of the stomach area.

In serious disease, with pain, you can safely leave the pack on for the whole of the three day period, taking the pack off only to shower. Then, of course, a three day period without the pack must be sustained.

It is recommended by all the famous healers that enemas be used during the period of castor oil pack use, so that the toxins which are released via the castor oil treatment will be expelled quickly.

Using the castor oil pack on the stomach area is helpful even if the cancer is not within this area, as digestion is improved, and toxins eliminated, which helps improve your digestive qi, increase energy flow, and improve your immunity. An improved immune system will help you in conquering the disease and recovering. The area with the cancer or other disease can be treated separately with another, separate pack which is of the size required.

When you have finished using the pack, put the pack into the storage container which you are going to keep specifically for your castor oil pack, so that it can be used again. Of course, eventually, you should replace the pack, especially if you are using it

frequently, but a castor oil pack should last for months when it is kept in an airtight container.

Note: Do not share the castor oil pack. One pack for one person is the motto. The one pack can be used many times over by the one person. Just keep adding a little more castor oil to it. Eventually you should discard the castor oil pack and make up a fresh one if you are using the three-day on, three-day off plan.

Chapter 5

Cancer Doctor's Treatment Uses Just Three Herbs

The Cure For All Cancers

This is the title of the book which Dr. Hulda Regehr Clark, Ph.D., N.D. wrote. In it she provides the details of her tried alternative cancer cure, which uses just three herbs for treating cancer. She has successfully used this herbal treatment over a period of many years.

Her recipe of wormwood or artemisia, cloves, and tincture made from black walnut hulls, is a traditional herbal mixture which Percy Weston also mentions in his book.

Of course, Dr. Clark recommends certain dietary changes, as well as lifestyle changes, and gives a list of numerous cancer-inducing chemicals which must also be avoided to combat cancer.

Dr. Clark has observed parasites of many varieties in the livers and intestines of all her cancer patients. She has also found isopropanol present in the livers of all the people she has treated for cancer. This chemical, which is found in cleaning fluids, cooling agents and some cosmetics, has an affinity for a common parasite which favours cancerous conditions, the Fasciolopsis buskii. This is a leaf-shaped intestinal worm, or fluke. This parasite can cause such conditions as Crohn's Disease, irritable bowel syndrome, colitis, and cancer, according to Dr. Clark. She maintains that if you get rid of this parasite, then you will get rid of cancer.

Walter Last had a similar belief – that it was an organism thriving in the intestines which was causing many health problems, including cancer.

The herbs which Dr. Clark uses can cure cancer parasites within five or six days. Continued treatment reduces cancer tumours, and also kills off other unwanted organisms which can take hold in the human body. 'Cancer can now be cured, not just treated', she claims.

She feels so confident of her method in curing cancer, that she warns against surgery to have organs removed, 'because you just might need them when you recover', she says.

Dr. Gerson had the same approach in keeping the vital organs. He refused to treat people who had undergone chemotherapy or radiation, as this damaged the organs and reduced the likelihood of recovery. Surgery, radiation, and chemotherapy are all best avoided if you opt for a recovery using natural methods.

There are several well-tried and proven alternative therapies for treating cancer. Dr. Hulda's is just one of them. I am well-acquainted with Dr. Gerson's castor oil /enema method for curing cancer, as well as those variations used by Walter Last, Dr. Ann Wigmore, and New Zealand's own natural-cure doctor, Dr. Eva Hill. Then there are all those practitioners of the Vitamin C Megadose and Laetrile treatments who have had amazing successes (read the later chapter in this book on Vitamin C and Cancer).

Dr. Hulda's cancer treatment is not one I have personally tried, but there is no doubt as to the efficacy of her method, since she has used it successfully over many years in her clinic.

I give it to you because of its simplicity. The method is straightforward and easy to understand, and it does not require that you purchase any strange or relatively unknown expensive herbs, or attempt any difficult procedures which some other treatments demand. It might be just the thing for people who are not familiar with alternative therapies for cancer and other diseases.

So, if you are contemplating surgery for cancer, then I would urge you to postpone the surgery, talk to your health professional about trying her method for a month, and then go back for a checkup to see if your cancer has reduced in size. Then you might have a better idea about whether you should take that surgery or not. Once your organs have gone, they have gone for good. If there is a way you can keep them, why not put in the time and effort to give it a go?

Quite recently, my sister's friend was diagnosed with optic nerve cancer. She was told by a specialist at the Auckland Hospital that she would need to have her eye removed within a month. She hated this idea, and went on her own programme of herbal treatment, with dietary changes and meditation, and now, only two months after beginning her own health regime, the eye cancer has reduced from 5.2mm to 3.6mm, all in the space of two months.

Dr. Clark includes one hundred case histories in her book which illustrate the effectiveness of her method. She includes a list of carcinogenic chemicals which you need to avoid in order to recover and stay well, and foods to avoid as well.

Dr. Clark waited until she had one hundred successful cancer case histories to report before publishing this book in 1993. She has since written another book entitled 'The Cure For HIV and AIDS'.

Dr. Clark's Three Herb Treatment For Cancer

The treatment is comprised of Black Walnut tincture, Wormwood combination capsules, and Cloves. All of these herbs are used every day for around three months. But each herb has a different dose, and is introduced in graduated doses, so read this carefully, and be sure to follow the instructions correctly.

1) How To Use The Black Walnut Tincture

On the first day of treatment, take just one drop of black walnut tincture. Repeat the dose of one drop four times during the day, just for the first day. It can be taken at anytime, morning or afternoon. Just divide the doses up so that they are spaced at least an hour apart. Dr. Hulda Clark advises to take the tincture half an hour before meals. It can be added to any healthful drink. Over the next three months, while doing this herbal treatment for cancer, avoid the use of coffee, tea or alcohol.

On the second day of treatment, the dose is increased to two drops of black walnut tincture, which is taken four times during the day as before.

On the third day of treatment, the dose is increased to three drops of black walnut tincture. As before, the same dose is repeated four times during the day. Keep on increasing the dose by one drop per day. Whatever you have increased the dose to, it is repeated four times daily as above, until you have reached twenty drops of black walnut being taken four times during the day.

It is very important to increase the dosage gradually, increasing by one drop per day as per instruction above. Do not be tempted to take a shortcut by skipping the graduations and using a large dose of black walnut to start with. This would shock your liver and your heart, and undoubtedly have an adverse effect. When you have gradually increased the dose up to twenty drops per day, the dose is immediately reduced the following day. You keep taking twenty drops in one go, one dose of twenty drops, but you use it only once a day.

From now on, only one dose is taken daily, using twenty drops of black walnut tincture to be taken in the one dose. This one dose is repeated daily for a period of three months.

Whilst using the Black Walnut tincture, as described above, you also take Wormwood in the form of capsules.

2) The Procedure For Using The Wormwood Combination Capsules

On the first day of treatment (as well as the specific dosage for black walnut as outlined above) take just one capsule of wormwood with a glass of water before the evening meal.

On the second day of treatment, double the dose of wormwood to just two capsules before the evening meal. Keep taking the black walnut tincture as described above.

On the third day of treatment, increase the wormwood capsules to one dose of three capsules, taken all in one dose, just before the evening meal.

The dose of wormwood is gradually increased by one capsule per day until you are up to fourteen capsules per day, which are still taken altogether just before tea time. By this time, concurrent with the wormwood treatment, you will also be taking just the one dose of the black walnut tincture each day.

When you have reached fourteen capsules of wormwood, continue with fourteen capsules for just two more days, one dose of fourteen capsules each day before tea.

At this point, the dose is suddenly dropped to a twice-weekly dose: fourteen capsules, which are still taken altogether in the one dose, are taken only twice a week. Leave a space of three or four days before taking the second dose of fourteen capsules.

From now on, you take keep taking the Wormwood twice a week indefinitely, using the same dose of fourteen capsules which are taken altogether .

Continuing this dose permanently prohibits parasites from re-entering your digestive system and vital organs.

3) The Procedure For Using The Third Herb, Cloves

On the first day of treatment, just one capsule of cloves is taken three times a day before meals.

Double the dose of cloves on the second day to two capsules. You will take two capsules of cloves on the second day three times a day, one dose before each meal.

On the third day, increase the dose to three capsules, which will be taken before each meal: that is three capsules taken three times a day. You will continue to take the specified doses of black walnut and wormwood as well, as described earlier.

For the next week, up until the tenth day, take the three capsules of clove powder three times a day, that is, three capsules before each meal, every day until day you reach day ten.

On day ten, the dose is reduced dramatically: You will take only one dose of clove powder capsules, using three capsules per day.

No more change to the clove routine for another three months: keep taking just three capsules per day, in the one dose before tea, for three months.

After three months have passed, reduce the dose of clove capsules to three capsules taken just twice a week. Select two days of the week for the taking of your clove capsules, for example, three capsules taken every Monday, and again three capsules taken every Friday.

Dr. Hulda Clark recommends that you continue taking three capsules of cloves twice a week 'forever', as well as the wormwood. This ongoing treatment kills off shigella and all other pathogenic organisms, and will prevent cancer-causing parasites from re-infesting your body ever again.

Chapter 6

Vitamin C And Cancer

Vitamin C Inhibits Cancer Cells

In June 2015, it was reported on National Radio that New Zealand research scientists had proved for a fact that Vitamin C does have an effect on cancer cells. Actually, they are not the first, as the Australian doctor, Dr. Goodhope, the American Dr. Levy, and others have been writing about their studies into the effectiveness of Vitamin C for many years now. There is a wealth of research which shows that Vitamin C can stop cancer from growing, that it can reduce the size of cancers, and that Vitamin C can prevent cancer from developing in the first place.

NOTE: Although I would take the alternative approach every time, readers should not necessarily follow my advice. Different things work for different people. DO see a doctor or a suitably qualified health professional if you think you may have cancer or some other degenerative disease.

The Vitamin C Debate

For years, the debate about Vitamin C and Cancer has continued, with some alternative health therapists using megadoses of Vitamin C to treat cases of cancer and other degenerative disease, whilst orthodox medicine stood outside the square insisting that their methods, which exclude the use of Vitamin C, were best.

The efforts and successes of the proponents of Vitamin C have largely been ignored, or minimised in many cases. Medical magazines are resistant to publishing material which is controversial. The power of persuasion of drug companies, and their readiness to stamp out opposition, are managing to keep the wonders of Vitamin C a big secret.
Using Vitamin C as part of a 'natural' treatment for cancer has been used for over 50 years. Dr. Max

Gerson, who used it in his famous cancer clinics, was driven out of America by the drug companies and the FDA, really because these powerful organisations did not want Dr. Gerson challenging the effectiveness of their drug and radiation methods for cancer, when his own methods were so hugely successful.
You can read Dr. Gerson's book, 'A Cancer Therapy: Results of Fifty Cases', to get greater insight into his work. The book by Samuel E. Epstein, 'The Politics of Cancer', gives many instances of drug coverups and how alternative practitioners such as Dr. Gerson have been hunted down and ostracised by the strong arm of the FDA, which is backed by the pharmaceutical companies.

Alternative therapies are kept such a secret, most people don't even consider a 'natural', or alternative cancer therapy when they first discover they have cancer. I met a woman at a public swimming pool recently, who was due to have her breasts taken off because of malignant breast cancer. I told her about the clinic in Remuera, Auckland, which gives intravenous Vitamin C for cancer and advised her to go there for advice before having the operation. 'Oh, I don't believe in Vitamin C. If it worked, then we would all hear about, and the hospitals would be using it,' she said. She was wrong. She believed implicitly in the medical system. She was not even mildly aware that modern medicine is one of the biggest industries in the world, or that the medical profession are basically puppets for the multinational drug companies, who refuse to accept alternative methods which could pose a threat to their monopoly on the health 'industry'.

Another recent major happening which should elevate the status of Vitamin C in treating any serious disease, also occurred very recently, again in

New Zealand.

The case, which has drawn attention to the media, is one where Vitamin C cured a case of swine flu and hairy cell leukemia. The man, who was in hospital, was not improving with the current regular methods of treatment. The family of the man requested that he be given Vitamin C in megadoses; they had read somewhere that this could be effective. However, the medics denied this treatment at first, saying that it would not do any good.

The family did not give up, and threatened legal action unless Vitamin C was administered before the man died. So the hospital authorities relented, gave the man the megadoses of Vitamin C, and the result is that the man recovered from Swine Flu and Hairy Cell Leukemia.

We had coverage on the case by reporters from Channel 3 and Channel 1, TVNZ, which was excellent.

I hope that the subject still remains 'hot' news, as it very well should be. So often, when major alternative 'findings' come to light here, they quickly get drowned by other competing factions, and are then conveniently forgotten: sometimes it is years before we have any more reporting on similar issues.

Lives could be saved if, as well as Vitamin C treatment, homeopathic medicine were at least given a try in some of these 'incurable' illnesses. Let's pray that the pharmaceutical companies loosen their strangulating hold on the medicine industry, and let Homeopaths prove the worth of their science, as well as the Vitamin C therapists.

See also http://merrilynhope.com/curing-the-incurable-with-vitamin-c/

Chapter 7

Intravenous Vitamin C For Cancer Offered At Private Clinic

Natural Remedies For Treating Cancer

Vitamin C is antiviral, antifungal, antibacterial, and acts as an antihistamine. It helps the body detoxify, which is why it is such a valuable remedy to use in cancer treatments.

Remember that, as with orthodox therapies, there is no guarantee that you will recover with Vitamin C and complementary therapies. However, mega-doses of Vitamin C, when continued over a period of time, have the ability to cure many cancers, or at least halt their development. Vitamin C has been recognised as a cancer inhibitor for a long time now. Taking Vitamin C intravenously means that mega-doses of the Vitamin can be given without the digestive system being affected. Up to 70,000 milligrams of Vitamin C can be safely administered in this way. The amount depends on the body weight of the person, and other factors. These large doses are often extremely effective, shocking cancer into remission. Vitamin C, taken in megadoses on a regular basis and combined with raw juices and detoxification measures such as castor oil and enemas, can gradually reduce cancer masses by killing off the cancer cells.

I have had experience with a clinic in Auckland, New Zealand, who give intravenous Vitamin C. Their address is directly below. If you live in America, or elsewhere, then try contacting The Vitamin C Foundation (www.vitamincfoundation.org). They have a lot of information on their website, and should be able to direct you to your closest Vitamin C clinic.

The address of the Auckland clinic is Integrated Health Options, 110 Remuera Road.
Phone New Zealand 09 5247743
Queries to their website:
info@integratedhealthoptions.co.nz

Two friends of mine have recently had successes with natural therapies for cancer – after reading my posts on the subject and listening to my raves, they decided to give the detoxification techniques a really good try.

One friend decided to have her ovaries removed for a start, the place where the cancer had begun. It was thought there were secondaries in other parts of her body also.

After the operation, she went weekly to the Remuera clinic for intravenous shots of Vitamin C. She also began a juice diet with plenty of fresh organic salads. About six to nine months later there is no sign of any cancer, according to her hospital specialists. Now that she is cured, they say she may not have had cancer anyway. Such is the reluctance of many medical professionals in accepting that some natural therapies, such as Vitamin C, do actually work.

The other friend, a male, had cancer of the pancreas. He lives in the country and does not have access to intravenous Vitamin C treatment. So he used plenty of non-acidic Vitamin C instead, calcium ascorbate, which has had the acid neutralised. I advised him to take up to 10,000mg per day, in doses of 1000mg at a time.

As well, his partner encouraged him to detox on raw juices and lots of salads. He was fortunate to have her help in preparing a nourishing raw food and juice diet.

He also took castor oil every second day for a few months. I had impressed the necessity for castor oil and enemas, as well as the Vitamin C, as he had looked so terrible. Many had expected he would die before long, as the hospital could do no more good for him. I suspect that he also did the enema-cleansing of the bowel as well, as his demeanour was so dramatically improved, but I thought it imprudent to ask.

It was great to see him smiling and looking so radiantly healthy when I met them again. It had been five months since I had last seen them, when they had both looked extremely ill and depressed. Now, they were both so very happy with the result of their efforts. They delighted in telling me the story of their victory over the illness which had nearly put him into his grave.

Note: The Longevity Foundation in Auckland may be able to help you source a quantity of affordable, quality Vitamin C.

Chapter 8

Vitamin C Cures Swine Flu Case

Massive doses of Vitamin C, administered intravenously, effected a cure of a dying man when drugs
were having no effect.

This very exciting healing event was documented
by TVNZ in 2010. Go to http://ondemand.tv3.co.nz
to view the documentary entitled: 'Vitamin C cures
case of swine flu and hairy cell leukemia'.

This is an amazing story, and it is wonderful for
the man and his family that this treatment has succeeded. The event should represent a breakthrough
in orthodox medicine which should bode well for
future usage of Vitamin C in our hospitals. But as
is usually the case, it is four years since Vitamin C
cured this man of swine flu, and no more has been
heard about his story, or the wonders of Vitamin C.
The hospitals are strangely silent, and doctors still
do no more than before to promote Vitamin C in
their treatments, at least in the town where I live.

This is because drug companies do not endorse the
use of Vitamin C, and insist on using their pharmaceutical drugs, even when it is clear they are not
working.

Why is this so? The answer is that Vitamin C is relatively cheap, as are homeopathic remedies, and is
a safe remedy or cure for many ailments. I believe
that if people were in the habit of using Vitamin C, or
homeopathy, there would be very little need for doctors, their drugs, or hospitals, except for emergency
situations such as accidents or surgery. Pharmaceutical companies would die a natural death.

The Benefits Of Vitamin C

The benefits of Vitamin C in treating disease have
been well researched. There is a wealth of literature
on the subject of Vitamin C and how it works as a
powerful antioxidant and detoxifier of the body, and
how it is an essential ingredient in treating cancer,
degenerative disease, and so-called incurable

infections such as swine flu.

High doses of Vitamin C are used in many alternative cancer treatment centres, in combination with other treatments. Therapists in Australia have successfully treated many people for swine flu, snake bites, and cancer with megadoses of Vitamin C. Vitamin C is really a wonderful nutrient.

But there is still much resistance to using Vitamin C in the medical profession. The man who survived swine flu was extremely lucky to have the support of a family who believed that the Vitamin C treatment could cure their brother. It was fortunate that they were present at the hospital at the time, to fight their brother's case.

Doctors at this Auckland hospital were determined, in the beginning, not to administer Vitamin C. They said that it would make no difference, and that it was against hospital policy. Medically speaking, there was absolutely nothing else they could do, and the man was about to die. Yet they still denied the man Vitamin C as a last resort.

But the family were adamant that Vitamin C treatment at least be tried. They had nothing to lose if the treatment did not work. Conventional medicine had failed. The medical staff were removing the life support system to leave the man to die, and the only hope left was that the Vitamin C treatment might work.

And so the family of the dying man threatened legal action if the medical authorities refused to administer Vitamin C.

The outcome of their efforts was that the authorities, under threat of being sued, finally relented and gave the intravenous Vitamin C as requested by the family. The quick result is what has been described as a 'miracle cure'.

I believe it is high time that some intelligent topics of research be chosen by so-called research scientists, such as the REAL reason for cancer and how diseases such as swine flu can be treated with Vitamin C. But this is unlikely to happen because of the power and wealth of drug companies.

If allowed to pursue an honest line of enquiry, I am certain that the majority of research scientists would find agreement with holistic medicine in recognising that cancer and other degenerative disease is a product of our toxic environment and the contaminated and devitalised foods which we eat.

They would acknowledge the healing effect of Vitamin C in healing cancer and so-called incurable diseases such as swine flu.

They might own up to the fact that there never will be a miracle pill to 'cure' cancer, but that cancer can be both prevented and reversed by positive strategies, mainly in adopting a remedial diet with detoxification techniques: That is, by eating good quantities of high fiber raw foods, and by purging toxic chemicals from the liver and intestines.

Using megadoses of Vitamin C in combination with other herbs and modalities encourages detoxification of a sick body, which gives it the chance, along with raw foods, to be revitalized and brought back to health. This is how you 'cure' cancer the natural way: by hard work and consistent effort.

Let's hope that Vitamin C is always available to the general public. The drive for profit often results in valuable, inexpensive, healing therapies being declared 'unsafe' by governments who have the backing of the multinational, powerful drug companies. Natural medicines which were previously readily available, such as gentian violet, have been taken off the shelves, and the same medicine then can now be sought only on prescription at grossly inflated prices, after we have also paid for the visit to the doctor to get the prescription. This red-tape for a prescription is designed to discourage us from using such cheaper remedies as gentian violet, and to buy off the shelf pharmaceuticals instead, which are comparatively more expensive for very small amounts. Whereas gentian violet keeps indefinitely, commercial skin creams have an expiry date, which means more cream has to be purchased before long. This is how profit is increased for pharmaceutical companies.

Lives could be saved if Vitamin C was used in combination with homeopathic medicine to treat so-called 'incurable' illnesses. Let's pray that the pharmaceutical companies loosen their strangulating hold on the medicine industry, and let Homeopaths prove the worth of their science, and the practitioners of Vitamin C therapy too.

Chapter 9

Dr. Eva Hill's Natural
Cancer Therapy

Raw Food: A Natural Remedy For Cancer

'Why Be Scared Of Cancer?' This is the title of Dr. Eva Hill's famous healing book which was published in New Zealand in 1979 by G.K. Moore. Her other book is 'A Simple Guide To Better Health', 1975.

Dr. Eva Hill, who was born Eva Day, is a famous New Zealand doctor who promoted a 'natural' cure for cancer. She helped save many lives through her alternative cancer therapy, and was convicted because of it, ironically enough, at the court in Christchurch where her father worked as a magistrate.

She had an uncle who was a doctor – this was the famous cricketer, W.G. Grace.

She was outstanding for her time, being one of the first women, and one of the youngest students, to graduate from the Otago University Medical School, in Dunedin, New Zealand.

Dr. Hill worked as a GP for many years, and entered politics in 1954. However, she developed cancer in an old wound in her cheek which changed the direction of her career.

Surgery on the cancer was not successful, and so she decided to follow a naturopathic treatment at the famous Hoxsey naturopathic clinic in Dallas, Texas. This treatment cured her cancer entirely.

Dr. Hill came back to New Zealand in 1956 and began to treat people using the 'natural' cure for all ills. Having cured her own cancer with a natural treatment, she was convinced that raw foods would cure most of her patients of their degenerative diseases, She believed that all cancers were treatable with raw foods, including malignant melanoma.

Eva Hill was an advocate for homegrown, organic food. She gave talks on the subject of growing organic food and how good nutrition was the key to preventing cancer and maintaining good health. She was a foundation member of the New Zealand Soil and Health Foundation.

She also campaigned against the fluoridation of

water, as she believed that this practice contributed to diseases like cancer.

The well-publicised success of her own cure, as well as the successes she was having with her patients, brought her under the spotlight of the medical profession and the powerful multinational drug companies who did their best to stop her practising as a doctor. They had already been alerted by Dr. Gerson's success in America as to the growing interest in natural treatments for cancer, and were determined to put a stop to practitioners of these treatments, especially if the practitioners belonged to the medical profession.

Dr. Max Gerson was targeted by the drug companies and the FDA in America, for using unorthodox methods of treatment for cancer. He was forced to stop practicing medicine in America, and so he set up his alternative cancer clinic in Mexico, where the American authorities had no sway.

Dr. Eva Hill was charged under the Health Act, N.Z., and was virtually convicted in court because of not using drugs in her treatments.

Dr. Hill appealed with the help of her supporters, and won her case. She continued with her natural healing methods, curing and helping untold people during the course of her career.

As a general rule for maintaining good health, she advised the avoidance of all animal proteins, all cereals, white sugar and salt. This is the same advice given by Walter Last, another prominent healer who worked in New Zealand a little later than Dr. Eva Hill. Walter also cured many people of their so-called terminal illnesses using natural remedies.

Method For The Eleven-Day Cleanse
Here is Dr. Eva Hill's method for an eleven-day cleanse, which she outlines in her book entitled 'Why Be Scared Of Cancer?'.

Epsom Salts Bath Each Night: One pound of epsom salts is added to the bathwater each night. This is continued for the first week of the treatment. Epsom salts draw out toxins from the skin and the tissues beneath. Magnesium from the salts is absorbed through the skin, which nourishes the body and helps remove acidity. It also stimulates the circulation.

First Three Days: Fast on water with citrus juice. Dr. Hill recommends a glass of grapefruit or orange juice every four hours. Nothing else is eaten or drunk during these three days except for water and citrus juice.

Next Two Days: Continue with the citrus drinks, but add fresh fruit to the diet also. Apples, grapes, peaches, pears, and tomatoes are all good. She says baked apple can be included at this stage.

For The Following Six Days: For breakfast have only fresh citrus such as grapefruit or oranges. Lunch is comprised of salad using from three to six fresh vegetables. Finish lunch with one cup of homemade potassium broth.
How to Make Potassium Broth: You can make a potassium broth by slowly stewing any green vegetables, or root vegetables. Do not add fruits to your potassium broth.
Use four or five vegetables in combination, such as chopped potatoes with their skins left on, provided the potatoes have not turned green, parsnips, kumara, pumpkin, carrots, onions, parsley, silver beet or spinach, kale, cabbage, or celery.
Cover the chopped vegetables with plenty of water and simmer gently for around an hour. Allow to cool, then drain off the liquid and keep in the fridge. Drink a glass frequently throughout the day.
Make a fresh potassium broth every three days and

throw out leftovers of the previous broth.

Dinner: Lightly cooked, or steamed vegetables, followed by another cup of potassium broth.

After-dinner snack: Make a salad of fresh sweet fruits. Remember that sweet fruits should not be combined with sour fruits. Sweet fruits such as bananas, feijoas, grapes, apples, peaches and nectarines can be used in any combination.

On Completion of the Cleansing Diet

After ending this cleansing diet and resuming a balanced one, Dr. Hill recommends continuing to take a glassful of fresh fruit juice daily before breakfast. Orange, grapefruit, apple, or grape juice, or an unsweetened lemon drink using the juice of one lemon. For breakfast make a fresh fruit salad using sweet fruits of any kind as listed above. Grated or ground nuts and honey can be included with the fruit.

Dr. Hill recommends that her elimination programme be repeated two or three times during the year to maintain good health. She also says to follow the programme whenever constipation or a cold or flu appears, or during any other illness where a fever is involved.

Chapter 10

How Doctors Used Homeopathy To Cure Fibroid Tumours

Homeopathic Remedies Which Have Been Used Successfully To Treat Fibroids And Other Tumours

Cancerous tumours are difficult to cure with medicines alone. Most alternative cures that I have come across, including my own modified diet which cured a breast lump years ago, have involved following a very strict but nutritious diet with rigorous cleansing measures.

See also about Vitamin C for Cancer:

http://merrilynhope.com/vitamin-c-and-cancer/

Cancerous tumours have been successfully cured by some doctors who used homeopathic treatments. It is probable that their patients' homeopathic treatment were combined with a specific healing diet, but if this were the case, the details are not given in my sources.

I have taken some examples of homeopathic healing for tumours from those given by Dr. Dorothy Shepherd in her book, entitled 'Magic Of The Minimum Dose: Impressive case histories by a world famous Homeopath' which was published by B. Jain Publishers in 1998.

Cancers take a time to develop, and it takes a time to reverse them again. As with other diet and cleansing methods for treating cancer, according to Dr. Shepherd and other doctors whom she quotes, the tumours treated with Homeopathic remedies also took around a year or two to disappear.

Sequence Of Homeopathic Remedies Used To Heal Uterine Fibroid Tumours

Homeopathic Sulphur 5 t.d.s was used by Dr. Shepherd to begin the treatment for fibroid tumours. She outlines the case of her patient with fibroid tumours on pages 84–85 of her book.

The patient had been diagnosed with fibroids by another doctor, and he had recommended her to have an operation. But on this revelation, instead of having an operation, the patient had decided to seek help from Dr. Shepherd and to try her homeopathic remedies to reduce the tumours naturally.

Dr. Shepherd's patient had many classic Sulphur symptoms: she had menstrual problems; she had been very constipated and was taking 'Normacol' to help the constipation. She was also suffering severe indigestion, bloating and flatulence and was taking baking soda regularly to help relieve the problem of acidity.

Other sulphur symptoms which this patient exhibited were shortness of breath, being the worse for exertion, disliking the fat of meats and cod liver oil, was worse in the morning around 11 a.m., and worse for summer heat. She also suffered pain in the mid-scapular region of the back, but felt better when lying down and resting.

The patient was given the Homeopathic Sulphur remedy as described.

Two months later the patient visited Dr. Shepherd again. Dr. Shepherd observed that she seemed much improved already. Her excessive menstrual period had reduced to only four days, her uterus was less inflamed than it had been on the previous visit, and she was experiencing less clotting of blood. Her indigestion had improved, although she was still taking the laxative which was not prescribed by Dr. Shepherd.

The patient at this point told Dr. Shepherd she had earlier been treated in a sanatorium for apical tuberculosis. Tuberculosis, even when it lies dormant in the genes for generations, can cause many health problems of the lungs, and of the reproductive organs. So Tuberculinum 30 was prescribed, to be taken once a week, four powders in each weekly dose.

As well, Dr. Shepherd prescribed Fraxinus americana 0 to be taken each morning and night, five drops each dose. Dr. Shepherd says that the renowned Dr. Burnett had cured many cases of fibroids with this Fraxinus remedy, which he described as an 'organ' remedy.

The patient went away with her homeopathic Tuberculinum remedy and her homeopathic Fraxinus. It was six months before she came back to see Dr. Shepherd. By this time her health was much improved, and she was not taking the laxative anymore.

She went back to the original doctor for a routine examination. This doctor observed that, since seeing the patient six months ago, the fibroids had almost disappeared with Dr. Shepherd's homeopathic treatment.

The patient continued with Dr. Shepard's treatment, the homeopathic Fraxinus o mins V remedy. She took it morning and night, as before, and did so for another eight months.

The fibroids had disappeared completely after this time, but nervous and mental symptoms which she had suffered in the past returned. The symptoms were fear of being alone, headaches before her period, and other symptoms which fit with the Nat. mur remedy.

Nat. mur was then given as a constitutional remedy to fix those general symptoms of stress.

Chapter 11

The Grape Cure
Used By Johanna Brandt

Alternative Treatment For Cancer: The Grape Cure

My dear friend, the healer and impressionist artist Bernhard Petersen, just loved grapes. He believed in their healing qualities so much, he let them grow in and around his house on Waiheke Island, Mediterranean style, all over the perspex ceiling of his studio and into parts of the living room. The grapes did well there. This dear friend taught us so much, and healed many people while he lived on Waiheke.

Grapes have been used in healing for thousands of years. People in Mediterranean countries commonly use grapes as a fasting measure, just as Bernhard did. They are rich in minerals and vitamins, and have a cleansing effect on the liver, the intestines, and the blood.

Grapes are a superfood food which can restore people to health.

Johanna Brandt cured herself of cancer by using grapes for a time. Walter Last believed in their health properties. Many other people have had success in healing with grapes.

Johanna Brandt's story is a remarkable one, and it serves as inspiration for the rest of us who wish to prevent or cure degenerative disease. She has written accounts of her own success, and the good results which followed when she began to treat other people with her grape diet.

Note: Not everyone who attempts a 'natural cure' will recover from a degenerative disease such as cancer. The information contained in this chapter is not an assurance that you will succeed. Many factors come into play when you are attempting to rid yourself of cancer.

If you or a loved one has cancer it may be helpful to ask the following questions:

Has the person had any chemotherapy or radiation

therapy? Having these treatments reduces your chances of recovering using natural means.

Has the person had any organs removed? Having organs removed reduces your immunity and weakens the body generally. You need to keep your vital organs. Having them removed drastically reduces your chances of gaining a 'cured' status.

Dr. Gerson did not accept patients who had had chemotherapy or radiation, because he believed their chances of recovery to be very small. But despite the prognosis, some people, with much determination, have succeeded in at least prolonging their lives, if not curing their cancers, by adopting a diet predominant in raw foods after chemotherapy and radiation. Much more effort is required to recover if your body's strength has been undermined through these aggressive orthodox measures.

Johanna Brandt was born in South Africa in 1876. There was a history of cancer in the family: her mother died of cancer in 1916, so when she began to experience pain in the left side of her stomach, she suspected cancer.

Fasting initially helped Johanna, but she found that when she resumed eating other foods, including some cooked foods, the cancer pain returned and the growth got bigger.

She battled with the tumour for nine years before she discovered the one food which did not encourage the tumour to grow: grapes.

Johanna cured herself of cancer using her grape method, and went on to help other people recover.

Note: It is recommended that only organic grapes are used for this diet.

Outline Of Johanna Brandt's Method
First Part Of The Grape Juice Diet

1) Johanna starts her diet with two to three days of fasting on only water. A warm water enema is taken daily during the fasting period, which has the added juice of one lemon.

2) After fasting for several days, drink one or two glasses of purified water, or boiled water, in the morning before your breakfast of grapes.

3) Half an hour after the drink of water, you can begin eating grapes.

4) Begin your grape breakfast at 8 a.m. and have more grapes every two hours throughout the day.
Note: Some other therapists recommend simply eating as many grapes as often as you like, at no set intervals. Whenever you feel hungry, you just eat more grapes. This was Bernhard's method for detoxification, as well as for enjoyment.

5) Johanna's method would use seven meals of grapes per day, with some eaten every two hours.

6) The grape diet can be continued from two weeks to two months.

7) Several pounds of grapes should be eaten daily with Johanna Brandt's method.

8) Chew the grapes well, seeds and all. If your stomach finds the grapes too acid in the beginning, then the skins may be removed. Eventually, when your stomach has improved, you should eat the whole of the grape with its skin and seeds.

9) Nausea, dizziness or stomach cramps which you might experience in the beginning are usually due to poisons being expelled from the liver and other parts of the body. In order for these poisons not to be reabsorbed as they pass through the intestines, it is important that you have at least one daily enema.

Enema: This can be a simple warm water enema, with half a teaspoon of sea salt. The Gerson therapy uses coffee enemas to clear toxins out of the liver, but with the grape diet, warm water with sea salt will suffice. Johanna suggests using the juice of a lemon in the enema instead of salt.

When the enema water being expelled is clear, and you feel that you are sufficiently detoxified, you can begin a modified diet. You might spend several weeks, or up to two months on the modified diet.

The Modified Diet

Adopt this phase of the programme after several weeks of eating only grapes. The modified diet still includes grapes, but other foods are introduced as well.

Begin breakfast at 8 a.m. with your grape meal. At 10 a.m. you may take another fruit. Choose only one variety of fruit, and eat it on its own. Eat your grapes by themselves in one meal at breakfast, and then choose another fruit to eat on its own at 10 am.

Meanwhile, you continue eating grapes every four hours.

At 2 p.m. you can use cottage cheese, soured milk, or yoghurt with your fruit. Nuts or almonds can replace the dairy foods if you wish. If you opt for milk or yoghurt, I would do as Percy Weston suggests and use only whole, raw, unpasteurised milk.

A meal of raw tomatoes and olive oil can be taken instead of fruit. This option can be used to replace any of the fruit meals for variety. Meanwhile, the emphasis on grapes continues, with a meal of grapes eaten at four-hourly intervals during the day.

Breakfast should consist entirely of grapes, just the same as before.

No cooked food is used in this part of the diet: only raw fruits are eaten, with the addition of either soy or organic dairy products and /or nuts and seeds.

The Final Stage Of The Grape Cure

After several weeks on the modified diet above, you can eat any raw fruit and vegetables of your choosing. Cooked food is introduced at this point: just one cooked meal of vegetables is taken per day.

Dried fruits are acceptable, as long as they are unsulphured and do not have other preservative added.

Vegetables to use during the final stage of the Grape Cure: green beans, green peas, runner beans, spinach, celery, tomatoes, cucumber, parsnip, lettuce, cauliflower, broccoli, squash, cabbage, carrots, beetroot, spring onion and chopped onions, kale, sprouted mung beans. Any of these can be eaten in salads, or in the cooked meal.

Johanna Brandt recommends that you do not combine raw and cooked foods. She suggests keeping to the raw for breakfast, having lightly cooked vegetables for lunch, and having a salad for tea with soured milk, or cottage cheese, or nuts or almonds.

Later on, she includes potatoes, or rice, bread, or oatmeal in the daily diet, but these carbohydrate foods are only introduced after you have recovered from the cancer.

In the case of any pain returning, then the raw fruit and vegetable diet should be resumed, with grape meals taken every four hours as before.

For your salads you can use any of the vegetables

which are listed above.

You can add chopped raw nuts, almonds, grated cheese or sour cream to your salad.

Lightly cooked , hard boiled, free range eggs can also be added to the salad.

Olive oil aioli dressing, with raw egg yolk and olive oil, is a healthful dressing to use. Lemon juice and olive oil is also good. Do not use commercial dressings, as these will have additives.

Mashed banana, or another fruit, with organic sour cream or olive oil or nuts can be taken for the evening meal.

A salad of simply tomatoes and olive oil, with a little chopped parsley, and spring onion, is very tasty and delicious. Tomato and olive oil are used in the second phase of the treatment, and it is a nice option to include during the final stage as well.

Chapter 12

Black Walnut For Restoring Tooth Enamel

Medicinal Herbs: Black Walnut As A Restorative Herb

The same restorative diets as those used for cancer, arthritis, Parkinson's disease, and multiple sclerosis have proven successful in many cases for restoring tooth enamel.

Often, people have discovered that their teeth have repaired themselves whilst following a strict dietary and cleansing regime to treat skin conditions, such as eczema or psoriasis.

The green hulls of the Black Walnut, Juglans nigra, have a great reputation for facilitating healing, including the regrowth of tooth enamel. See Chapter 5 which outlines a traditional recipe for using black walnut tincture in healing cancer. This formula has been used with great success by Dr. Hulda Clark.

Louise Tenney, who wrote the book 'Today's Herbal Health', 1983, gives a summary of the healing attributes of the black walnut, in which she includes its ability to heal tooth enamel.

Valuable Minerals In Black Walnut

Here are some of the attributes of black walnut, as specified by Louise Tenney:

Black Walnut Husks and Leaves are rich in important healing minerals. Organic iodine, magnesium, manganese, Vitamin B15, silica, iron, calcium, potassium and phosphorus are all to be found in Black Walnut.

Iodine has antibacterial, and antiviral qualities. This is why Black Walnut, which has high levels of organic iodine, can be very helpful for the preservation of the teeth and the restoration of tooth enamel. Silica is another important mineral which helps to keep harmful germs at bay, as well as having an important function in building strong teeth, bones, hair and nails. Silica is found in the Black Walnut husks and leaves, as well as in Comfrey, Stinging Nettles, and Prickly Ash, which make all these herbs excellent for keeping teeth and gums healthy.

Comfrey is one of the richest sources of silica, which is a good enough reason to have the plant brought back for the general public to use again. Some countries banned comfrey because the drug companies convinced governments that it can cause cancer and should be banned. But some believe this was really so that they have the monopoly on all the healing ingredients contained in comfrey. Now that their research scientists have bred a comfrey which is devoid of the main cell-proliferant, allantoin, comfrey has suddenly appeared in our plant shops again, after being absent for ten years or more. But this hybridised comfrey is not as beneficial to the teeth, hair, bones or nails as the common garden variety, since it does not contain allantoin, and is low in silica.

Stinging nettles are another rich source of silica, but commercial herbicides and people's desire to control our roadside verges have almost caused extinction of this valuable healing plant.

Avoid Chemicals, Including Food Additives

Of course, it is not enough to simply use black walnut tincture, or another healing herb, on a daily basis. For Black Walnut tincture to be effective on the teeth, one needs to adopt the optimum nutritious diet, with plenty of protein, green vegetables, and plenty of raw salad material to keep the teeth clean and the saliva alkaline. The same applies for using Comfrey in the diet, or Nettles, or Prickly Ash rubbed onto the gums and teeth: you need to be following a sound and healthy diet, rich in green vegetables both raw and cooked, with adequate protein, and little or no sugary foods, for the teeth to restore themselves. You also need to avoid any harmful chemicals such as those food additives which are put into all sorts of

packaged food these days.
Even commercial breads contain preservatives which are very bad for the teeth as well as the general physical, mental and emotional states.

Cleansing With Castor Oil

Periods of cleansing, where raw foods are eaten for a day, or several days, and castor oil is taken on occasion, depending on the advice of your health practitioner, can be helpful in removing toxins from the body. Ridding the body of toxic chemicals, and avoiding contact with chemicals, can help the general health as well as the health of the teeth. Jacqui Davison grew new tooth enamel when she followed the cancer-cure outlined by Dr. Max Gerson, who cured many people of cancer during his lifetime. Castor oil was one of the most important ingredients of his cancer cure. He advised his patients to take Two tablespoons every second day. Castor oil used in this way is a powerful detoxifier and healing agent. Jacqui followed her healing diet with its rigorous cleansing procedures for almost a year before she realised that her teeth had repaired themselves. Healing of the teeth takes as long as it takes to heal an invasive cancer, and it requires the same amount of vigilant effort.
The following chapter gives more information on diets which have worked to grow new tooth enamel.

Chapter 13

Regrow Tooth Enamel And Strengthen Gums

Here is a summary for anyone interested in working on diet to help the condition of the teeth.

It takes a while to regrow tooth enamel, so you have to be prepared to follow the programme for at least six months. My child's tooth enamel repaired itself after 9 months on such a programme.

Many years ago, a friend came to me for advice about her teeth. The health of her teeth recovered completely after only three months on the diet.

However, in this case, the tooth enamel itself was not the problem, but her diseased gums. She was told by a dental specialist that she had an incurable disease and would lose all of her teeth if she did not have them all removed one by one and scraped. Each tooth was going to cost $5,000 to fix. She was worried because she would have to mortgage, or sell her house, to afford the dental work.

She decided to follow my diet to the letter. After three months of putting all her energies into the diet, her gums were healed. She went back to the dentist to show him the result. He said diet could not have had anything to do with her teeth, and that there couldn't have been anything wrong with her teeth in the first place. But it was he who had diagnosed an incurable gum disease several months before.

Of course, there are multiple ways in which you can improve the health of your gums and strengthen tooth enamel. Here is just one suggested method, which is similar to the method I advised my friend to follow in order to heal her gums.

The Key Points Of The Diet To Regrow Teeth
Remove sugar, dairy foods and wheat altogether.
Stay gluten free: Instead of wheat pasta and bread, use brown rice. Avoiding gluten is important.
Avoid vinegar and other fermented foods. No alcohol. No sauces such as tomato sauce, or soy sauce. It

is important to avoid fermented foods, as well as gluten, dairy and sugar, because these foods feed candida, or yeast infection. Candida albicans is the source of many problems with health, including poor gums and teeth.

No preservatives.

Eat plenty of raw celery and carrots. This is a key factor in regrowing your tooth enamel and improving the health of your gums. End each meal with these. This improves digestion, as well as the health of the teeth.

Keep the mouth alkaline. Chew a stick of celery after each meal to keep the mouth alkaline. Celery is a natural germicide and antibiotic which will keep germs at bay. Celery will help to discourage the growth of damaging bacteria which cause decay.

Celery is well known for its ability to help build strong bones. It helps to build strong teeth as well.

Celery is a high fiber alkaline food. Eating raw celery, and carrots too, helps to provide plenty of fiber for your digestion. Your intestines will be cleansed by eating these raw foods, which means that they will process your foods more efficiently.

Eat as much of your food raw as you can. Begin sprouting mung beans and alfalfa at home. Mung bean sprouts and alfalfa sprouts are especially alkaline. These clean the teeth as well, keep the mouth alkaline, and provide more fiber for the bowel.

All protein foods are OK. Eating meat will not do your teeth any harm as long as you eat enough alkaline salads and cooked greens to go with it. Generally speaking, high quality protein is good for those on anti-candida diets. Protein eaten with raw foods will help your teeth to grow. If you are vegetarian, then make sure your protein is adequate: supplement with plenty of sprouts, nuts and seeds and pulses. Ground sesame seed is especially good as it is rich in calcium.

Organic free range eggs are excellent. Try to eat two free range egg yolks each day. This is very nourishing for the body and easy on the digestion. You can include these with your olive oil dressing for your salad, or put them into a smoothie such as a banana smoothie with almonds, sesame or sunflower seeds. Two raw egg yolks per day is recommended for vegetarians.

Use plenty of sesame seeds and sunflower seeds, and coconut milk, especially if you are on a vegetarian diet. These are all very high in calcium and essential fatty acids.

All raw and cooked vegetables are good.

As Walter Last insisted, always eat something raw with every meal.

Rinsing the mouth out with coconut milk after each meal is helpful. Swish the coconut milk around for several minutes to eliminate harmful bacteria and help remove plaque.

It takes a while to notice the effects of such a programme, especially to regrow tooth enamel. If you really put the effort into following this diet, and faithfully exclude wheat, dairy, sugar, and yeasts, then you should see some positive results on your general health after about three months. If you were to continue on for another six months beyond that, you should see your tooth enamel beginning to repair itself.

Calcium Ascorbate Powder

This is a non-acidic form of Vitamin C which helps keep the body alkaline. It also kills bacteria and works as a potent digestive which maximizes your vitamin and mineral intake from the food you eat. It helps to detoxify the body.

Calcium Ascorbate was used in treating my friend's gum problem. My family also used this quite fre-

quently, which would have helped my child to re-grow tooth enamel. You need to take 1000 mg at least once or twice per day.
The non-acidic form of Vitamin C will not erode your tooth enamel.

Castor Oil Treatment
People on cancer diets who have regrown their tooth enamel have used castor oil as part of their treatment. The Gerson diet for treating cancer uses 2 tablespoons every second day, with enemas to flush away toxins quickly from the bowel.
I think that taking castor oil even once a week will have a beneficial effect on your teeth. However, if the person is young, or healthy, with a strong recuperative power, regrowing tooth enamel can be done without castor oil.

Chapter 14

Toxic Dentures

The Cost Of Dental Treatment: Are Dentures A Good Option?

My, oh my, how I wish I had listened to Walter Last when I began following his dietary and detoxification measures: This was when I was very young, in my mid twenties, and I had only just discovered Walter and his diet. At that stage, I was simply following his advice in the hope that the diet would help me to recover from 2,4,5-T poisoning which had resulted in a breakdown of health, especially after my daughter, who was exposed to the chemical in the womb, had died. My teeth were the last of my concerns.

I had not read anything at all, at that stage, about the possible remarkable effects of the diet which Walter Last proposed on teeth regrowth.

I told Walter that I was thinking of having all my teeth removed, because at that stage we could not afford the expensive treatment required.

What I know now was that an inadequate diet with no dental care, and chemical poisoning to boot, had caused my teeth to suffer badly. A period of heavy alcohol use in my teens had probably not helped the condition of my teeth either.

Walter said I should just continue with the diet, and use herbs such as prickly ash on the teeth in the meantime. He assured me that things would get better.

But I did not listen. I had all my teeth extracted within several months of having my third child, just after beginning Walter's treatment.

I have paid dearly for this decision. Since this time, I have read a lot more and have learned about the successes of people like Jacqui Davison, who grew new teeth as she strived to beat cancer through diet and detoxification.

I have used a similar programme to Dr. Gerson's and Walter Last's to cure myself of a breast-lump, and to cure someone of serious gum disease which would have otherwise cost the woman the price of her house to fix, had she followed her dental specialist's advice, which was to submit to a removal and scraping operation on each individual tooth.

Toxins In Dental Plastic Plates

Dentures have a limited life. They become unhealthy because of toxins which are leached from the plastic and the epoxy resin glue which holds them together. I found no problem with the way they fit, the way they look, or the way they work in chewing food. It is the poisons in the plastic which I cannot abide. Toxins in the plastic are released as the plastic ages, and this causes major health problems for me, simply because the physical body is being 'fed' a constant supply of denture toxins on a daily basis. Consequently, I have needed new dentures every three years or so. Even with new dentures, and the most modern of denture plastics, the problem has not been entirely solved.

Unfortunately, taking antioxidants such as Vitamin C, or ginger, cinnamon, tea tree oil, eucalyptus, or garlic, can all have a counter-productive result when you have plastic in your mouth. This is because these herbs and vitamins, which all work to help remove poisons from the body, also have an effect on the plastic fabric of the denture. They cause poisons in the plastic to be released more readily. You can end up with toxic poisoning from the plastic of your denture if you use these items often.

Herbicides, Pesticides, Parabens: These All Affect Denture Plastic

Coming into contact with herbicides, pesticides and other chemicals such as parabens and isopropyl used in some toothpastes and cosmetics, also cause the denture plastic to behave in an extremely toxic way. Toxic chemicals get absorbed into the plastic, where they intensify the already toxic nature of the denture plastic. The result is a toxic cocktail of chemicals and, probably, pathogens.

Apple Moth Eradication Programme In Auckland

 When MAF were spraying Aucklanders with their 'apple moth' spray around the years 2001-2005, I was more ill than most people, because I was certain that this spray accumulated in the plastic of the dentures, and I simply could not get rid of it. This affected my whole health, including memory and even the ability to speak.

Just how and why our government and health authorities could justify using this spray all over the city for such an extended period is unfathomable. I am still curious as to their motives for using this spray which had an extremely deleterious effect on the health of so many people. We were not told the truth about the effects of the apple moth spray. Its ingredients were kept secret, except for its 'natural' soya base.

The spraying programme did not eradicate the apple moth. But it did have the effect of getting large amounts of the population going to the doctor for all sorts of mysterious illnesses, which must have boosted drug companies' revenue enormously, as well as the pockets of Auckland doctors.

One elderly friend, who moved into a house beside a stream of a valley which was being regularly aerially sprayed with the apple moth poison, became seriously ill within weeks of living there. His blood pressure soared. He went to hospital where one leg was amputated, and then the other was removed, and then he died.

Around this time, I had to throw away the current dentures which were only two or three years old, because they became incredibly toxic due to absorbing apple moth poison. This is just one cost I suffered, which, of course, was not reimbursed by MAF and their doctor. The other was that I had to suddenly quit living in the city, give away my piano teaching business and all household appliances like fridge, washing machine, and so on, and escape to the countryside. Otherwise, I am sure that my fate would have been similar to that of my friend who had died. About six or seven years ago, I found a new dental technician whom I thought had the answer for me. I paid $2,500 and a bit more at the time to get a fantastic new set of dentures which looked wonderful and were almost as good as my original teeth in their chewing function. This was the first set of teeth which I bought from this dentist.

A supposedly less-toxic and more expensive type of clear nylon fabric was used, with porcelain teeth, to minimise the amount of plastic in the mouth.

However, these teeth only lasted two or three years before the health issues began again. By the time two more years had passed, there was no doubt at all that the dentures were again undermining my health dramatically. Suddenly, one day, I could not stand them in the mouth any longer, as they were causing erosion of the mouth and lip tissues. My digestion was affected equally badly: it felt as if the same erosion and subsequent bleeding was occurring throughout the body. I took the teeth out, and recovered within a few days. I could not wear those teeth again, as every time I used them, the same symptoms would occur.

Health Problems From Dentures

Poisoning symptoms which I experience from these dental plate toxins include:

Breathing difficulty, breathlessness when walking quickly, amnesia and loss of memory, pains in the joints which developed into a weakness and paralysis if I continued to wear the dentures, plus earache, sinusitis, eczema, and poor vision.

Read my website article for more on this:
http://merrilynhope.com/burning-mouth-syndrome-from-dentures/

Because I had just turned 61, most people, including doctors, would say, 'You can expect these things to happen when you get older'. But the problem is not related to age, as I have been experiencing the same symptoms because of denture plastic for much of my life. And every time, no matter what my age has been, when the dentures are done away with, my health has immediately gotten much better. New dentures, except for one lot which were made of especially toxic plastic, and which I had to discard right away, tend to hold their toxic poisons intact for several years before they begin to break down and cause problems with health.

New Dentures Which Only Lasted One Year

Once I was completely sure about the bad effect of the dentures on my health, I went back to the same dental technician to have a brand new set made at the cost of $3,000.

Unfortunately, the life of this plate was reduced dramatically because the dentist mucked up the first moulding of the teeth. I am sure that he was angry because I said that denture plastic was causing ill health, which was why I was back to have another set of dentures made. He refused to take my story seriously, and told me I was not cleaning my teeth enough. He did not understand that copious cleaning, using products which he had recommended, had made the teeth even more toxic.

So, it seemed this dentist made very little effort in constructing my new dentures, due to our disagreement. He did a very bad job. They looked terrible, and he failed to align the top denture to the lower denture in the first moulding of the teeth. There were even two teeth missing on the lower denture which had been there on the previous denture. This meant there was no 'bite', as the two sets of teeth did not fit together.

I returned soon after, to get the matter put right, as I could not eat anything with these new dentures. It was through returning to this dental clinic, because of their initial error, that confirmed my belief about the hydroscopic nature of soft and malleable modern denture plastics, their potential for absorbing chemicals, and how vulnerable they are to heat. It was the effect of heat breaking down the fabric of the plastic which ultimately shortened the life of the teeth for me.

The faulty teeth had to be heated up to be remoulded again. It was this heating process which caused the immediate leaching of plastic chemicals into my stomach. From that day on, I had a permanent taste of glue in my mouth, and I was on the verge of collapsing. My brain would not function normally, my speech suffered, my tongue was swollen and I had pins and needles in my legs, arms and hands. But when I removed the teeth, all these symptoms would disappear within a very short time.

After experimenting for several weeks, there was no doubt that these new teeth were also causing harm to my health, just as the old ones had. I knew I should simply remove the teeth, swallow my pride and get used to a toothless image. But I had just paid $3,000 for them, and could not bear the idea of going about with no teeth. I battled with the problem of my pride, and the toxic teeth, for another 10 months. I got into the habit of wearing the teeth only on occasion, when I went out.

Why do dental technicians use such toxic materials as soft, hygroscopic plastic, when they could use a harder material which does not absorb poisons, or leach chemicals so readily? The reason is economics, as is the case for many products of questionable safety. If the dental technician makes an error with the first moulding, then they do not need to throw away the teeth to make a new set. Soft malleable plastic saves the dental technician money, because they can reuse this type of plastic. They simply heat the plastic up and remould the teeth.

This is an extremely unsafe practice, as heating up the plastic causes the leaching out of very toxic chemicals such as epoxy resin, formaldehyde, heavy metals and other poisons, all of which have the capacity to cause cancer, arthritis, and, in my experience, loss of memory. As far as I know, there is nothing organic or user-friendly about the chemicals commonly used in modern denture plastic.

This is ultimately the reason why I had to eventually throw these dentures away, as I explain below.

Suddenly, after ten months, the teeth became too toxic to wear. The taste of glue with the coolness of formaldehyde, or similar, became very intense, and the tissues of my mouth and lips were breaking down. I developed blisters on the lips and tongue. I could barely remember what I had been doing five minutes before, let alone remember people's names. I guessed it was the formaldehyde from the glue.

Formaldehyde has a disastrous effect on the memory and on brain function, as I had already experienced as a child. In hospital, after an operation for peritonitis, I had the unfortunate experience of having a thermometer come directly from a glassful of formaldehyde and thrust into my mouth several times a day. This caused a white-out, a complete blank in the brain. Then, when I recovered a little, shapes were distorted and I was very disoriented. Then, when the nurses came around again to take my temperature, the same would happen all over again. It was frightening, as I thought I would lose my mind completely if I was subjected to the hospital treatments much longer.

I feel sorry for the unwitting nurses who were handling thermometers in formaldehyde liquid every day. I read a newspaper article sometime in the 1980's, about two nurses of the period who had to leave the profession early because of chronic memory loss, and loss of concentration. They attributed their condition to formaldehyde exposure.

So now, fifty years later, I was experiencing similar symptoms to these nurses. The dentures were also causing pins and needles in the arms and hands, blurred vision, memory loss, chronic stomach pains, and other symptoms of poisoning.

No amount of cleansing or detoxifying agents could fix the problem of leaching chemicals.

I realised that the teeth had to go, and I would have to remain toothless if I was to retain the ability to think and live a meaningful life. There was no other way to avoid being contaminated by the poisons in this soft, malleable, denture plastic.

The denture plastic, apart from having been ruined by being heated up at the dentists to be remoulded, had also reacted to my using a quantity of tea tree oil which I had put on my hair and on my skin. Ironically, this was used to try and clear a sudden attack of eczema, which most probably was caused by the leaching of formaldehyde and parabens from the denture plastic.

I have found that tea tree oil, eucalyptus oil and other such strong embrocations are readily absorbed, just as toxic herbicides and pesticides are, into the denture plastic, and this causes the denture plates to erode more quickly, and leach even more chemicals out.

I had already noticed this in previous years with other dentures, that my dentures, which I was already becoming doubtful about with regard to their effect on my health, were made infinitely worse once tea tree or eucalyptus oil had been used. This would not be a problem if hard, stable plastic were used in the making of dentures.

So, let this be a warning to those people who consider that having false teeth might be a cheaper way to go. It has not been cheaper for me having dentures. If several sets only were needed during a lifetime, and they were not made of toxic material, then dentures would be a fine thing.

At the time of writing, I know of no safe alternative to the soft, malleable, porous, hygroscopic plastic which is currently being used for the making of dentures.

This type of denture is, in my experience, very bad for the health. The soft plastic which is being used in dentures could be one reason why so many people suffer Alzheimer's disease. We absorb too much plastic poison from other products in our environment, like having milk in plastic, plastic wrapping over meats and cheese, etc

But wearing plastic in your mouth has to be the very worst thing, because you are constantly absorbing a certain amount of poisons from the plastic into your system.

Until I can get a plate made which is not made of soft, porous plastic–something like the hard old thing which the soldiers in the second world war were fitted with–I will not wear dentures again.

My Dad has had an army-supplied plate for years, since 1943 when he went to war. I think he is still wearing the same one today. These old plates, although probably still made of toxic substances, should be better for the health because they are made of a stable, non-porous plastic. Hard, stable plastic does not absorb chemicals into its fibre, as soft plastic does, and nor does hard plastic leach chemicals so readily. It also has more resistant to heat, for obvious reasons.

In summary, I believe soft denture plastic can be very hazardous to the health. Plastic deteriorates, which means that, for your health's sake, dentures need to be replaced frequently. The cost of replacing dentures every few years is considerable, so think twice before having your teeth removed.

Chapter 15

Homeopathic Arsen Alb. As A Preventative And Cure For Flu

Arsen alb. in homeopathic dosage is considered by most reputable homeopaths to be a prophylactic for the flu. See the book by Dr. James H. Stephenson, 'A Doctor's Guide To Helping Yourself With Homeopathic Remedies' (1976).

I used homeopathic Arsen alb. with great success when flu was rife in New Zealand in 2013. I do not believe in vaccination. Apart from the possible side effects of vaccinations, they do not always work. See my writeup on the death of a vaccinated girl:
http://merrilynhope.com/vaccinated-nz-girl-dies-from-meningococcal-disease-3rd-september-2012/
Some of my friends who got flu injections still got the flu, and became very sick. I believe they would have had better results if they had used homeopathic Arsen. alb as a prophylactic and as a treatment for the flu.

Physical Symptoms Indicating Arsen Alb.

The patient needing Arsen alb. is usually thirsty, but only wants small sips of drink at a time. She feels chilled and needs warmth, except for the head, which is often burning. The skin is cold and often sweaty and clammy to the touch. The may be a severe headache when Arsen alb. is needed. 'Irritable, restless and discouraged' best describes the Arsen alb. patient. A cough or sore chest may go with any of the above symptoms.

Kent's 'Materia Medica', a widely studied text-book on homeopathy, indicates Arsen alb. for some forms of Asthma.

It is also a valuable remedy for some types of food poisoning. If one suspects food poisoning, homeopathic Arsen alb., taken every 15 minutes for six doses, can often avert the sickness which can result from eating tainted food.

Mental Symptoms Indicating Arsen Alb. Might Include

Feelings of extreme sadness, depression, wanting to die, mental anguish and anxiety. Wanting to avoid people because of a fear you have offended them in some way goes with Arsen alb. Ongoing sadness is one of the classic symptoms of the Arsen alb. patient.

Arsen Alb. Instead Of Flu Vaccinations

There are several very good homeopathic remedies which can be used as a prophylactic for flu, as well as a medicine to treat it. It may be that Arsen alb. is not the right one for you, in which case you could try another of the remedies, to find one which suits your constitution. But, since Arsen alb. is one the most commonly prescribed remedies, it is very likely that you will have some success with it.

It could be that, eventually, the medical profession endorse the use of Arsen alb. Flu vaccinations, as with many vaccines today, are very dubious in their effect. I do not believe in having vaccinations for flu. They are risky, and they do not always work in preventing the disease for which they are intended to protect. I prefer to use homeopathic Arsen alb., which is perfectly safe, poses no ongoing risk to the health, and has worked every time I have used it, either to prevent flu, or to facilitate a quick recovery.

A friend of mine, who lives in the same neighborhood as I do, went along for her flu vaccination recently, to prevent getting the flu which was of epidemic proportions. Three weeks afterwards, she got a 'bad' dose of flu. The injection made no difference, and she succumbed to the flu anyway. I probably caught the flu from this friend who had been immunised, but never mind. My homeopathic Arsen alb. came to the rescue.

I believe that you are more likely to suffer cancer, arthritis, multiple sclerosis, diabetes, obesity, depression, and/or a range of other diseases if you are in the habit of getting immunised.

Another friend of mine, who lives in the same street, can no longer have flu injections, because of severe and life-threatening allergic reactions which the flu vaccination caused. Three or four years ago, she had one injection which caused no problems. But the following year, just before holidaying in Australia, she had another flu vaccination which almost caused her death. Apparently the vaccination components had been changed from the one she had been given the previous year. She not only developed the flu immediately after this inoculation, but intense allergic reactions which, by the time they got to Australia, eventuated in her being hospitalized there in an intensive care facility. Their holiday was ruined, and so was her health, which she has had to build up very carefully since this vaccination disaster.

How Influenza Strengthens The Immune System.

I have just had a 'good' dose of the flu.

I welcome the flu each season, as it flushes out the system and kills off other organisms which might otherwise sap your energy. The fever which comes with the flu is actually a very beneficial thing which helps your body to throw off all the toxins it has been harbouring. The flu symptoms generally take away your appetite, which is another good thing in that you get to do a natural fast while you are recovering from the flu bug. Many toxins get expelled through having the flu, or diseases such as measles. This is a good thing, to expel poisons which might otherwise encourage a cancerous condition, if they were left in your body.

This attack of flu which I have just recovered from

without antibiotics or flu injections, responded very well to homeopathic Arsen alb., 30X. I did not need to use anything else in order to recover quickly from this flu virus of May, 2013. All I did was to keep taking regular doses of homeopathic Arsen alb., and keep warm. I also fasted for a week, taking only a little fruit or lemon drink to sustain me most days. During the first two days of this flu, my headache was chronic and almost unbearable. I took around five drops of Arsen alb. as needed, which was sometimes every 15 minutes, or half-hourly. As the headache and fever subsided, I reduced the dosage of Arsen alb. to three doses per day. Then, after a week, to around two doses per day. Then, after around ten days, to one or two doses per day to ensure no residual cough would remain.

Homeopathic Arsen alb. worked miracles for me. Often, after the flu, I get bronchitis which can take some time to recover from. This time, with just Arsen alb., I have recovered very quickly, and with very little bronchitis. Arsen alb. is also an effective cure for bouts of post-flu coughing.
I put down my quick recovery this time not just to the homeopathic Arsen alb., but to the lovely warm home which I now live in. A year ago I was living in a concrete basement flat which received no sun, and which was exposed to incessant winds off the sea. My health whilst living in this concrete, sunless flat, was very poor. I succumbed to the flu several times whilst living there, and never really got over the bronchial symptoms until I moved.

Alternatives To Vaccination For Flu
Arsen alb. is a natural antibiotic and cleanser of the system. It helps encourage elimination of toxins through the bowel, and helps cleanse the liver and other organs at the same time. Of course, I cannot say how well it would work on some of those new

and deadly strains of flu, but if it were me, I would be prepared to give homeopathic Arsen alb. a go, as well as some megadoses of Vitamin C, if I could get it. After all, as discussed in the previous chapter, Vitamin C megadoses have proved effective in curing some cases of swine flu.

Remember to stop taking your chosen remedy once you have really started to improve. Sometimes you can continue a treatment for too long, which can bring about a mimicking of some of the original symptoms. Thuja follows well after Arsen alb., and is a good remedy to antidote Arsen alb. if you have continued taking Arsen alb. for longer than necessary.

Chapter 16

Homeopathy And Vitamins For Mumps, Measles And Chickenpox

Alternatives To Vaccination: Homeopathy And Vitamin C

Of course, you must take your child to see a doctor or homeopath or naturopath if your child has a fever, or you suspect an illness. Here are some remedies which you and your health professional may like to consider to support treatment.

Homeopathic remedies work well when the right ones are given. With the help of a homeopath you can work out the right remedy for your child to treat any of the common childhood illnesses.

The information given below might be useful in an emergency situation, and to help if you choose not to vaccinate your child.

I believe it is a healthy thing for children to get measles, mumps and chickenpox. I chose not to vaccinate, and used homeopathic medicine instead.

It is my belief that getting these illnesses strengthens the child's immune system, and a strong immune system will help prevent them getting serious diseases such as cancer later in life.

Sometimes we hear about an unvaccinated child who suffers secondary afflictions from a childhood illness, and sometimes, they die. But these cases are not the norm in children who have not been vaccinated, at least not in children who have been treated with homeopathy.

Modern medicine has its failures: People often get the very sickness which they have been vaccinated for, and some have died after vaccinations. There is even a term for doctor-caused, drug-caused, or hospital-caused illness, which is Iatrogenic illness.

There are so many unknown hazards in today's world which can undermine your immune system, but vaccination is one potential risk which you can definitely rule out, by not doing it.

As long as the child has been properly nourished before getting sick, and is nurtured during these illnesses, then the child will generally do well to recover with the help of lemon drinks, homeopathy and vitamin treatment.

Measles, mumps, chicken pox, and, in fact, all the common childhood illnesses, can be dealt with effectively and safely with the use of homeopathy and/or vitamins and blue lighting.

And it is very interesting to note that even UNICEF has finally recognised the value of Vitamin A in treating measles. In 2013 Unicef gave out quantities of Vitamin A for an epidemic of measles in Syria. See my writeup http://merrilynhope.com/unicef-gives-vitamin-a-for-measles-in-syria/

I think that it is only a matter of time before homeopathy will again be used to combat outbreaks of measles, mumps and chickenpox, no matter where these epidemics arise. Antibiotics are losing their efficacy nowadays: Many diseases have become resistant to antibiotics. Swine flu, (pandemic H1N1), which struck in 2009 is one case in point. It could not be treated with antibiotics. Wikipedia reports 19,633 deaths out of 1,632,258 confirmed cases worldwide, until the point when WHO recommended that countries stop issuing data on the numbers affected.

In Australia and New Zealand, Vitamin C came to the rescue in several cases when it was administered in time, although not without much argument with hospital doctors, who said using Vitamin C was against hospital policy.

Homeopathy suffers the same resistance as Vitamin C in today's medical environment. Over one hundred years ago, homeopathy was very popular in Europe and America. It had been used successfully in Moravia to stem an outbreak of cholera, which did much to popularize homeopathy as a medicine in the UK and America in the early 1900's.

Homeopathic hospitals and teaching schools were set up in many places, the most notable of which was the Royal London Homeopathic Hospital, which was established in 1849. The Royal family were firm advocates of homeopathy. Unfortunately, the Royal London Homeopathic Hospital is no longer: It was subjected to a name change in 2010, and is now called the Royal London Hospital For Integrated Medicine. This must be a triumph for the historical opponents of homeopathic medicine.

As the drug companies in America got stronger, which was early on in the 20th century, they grouped together to form what was to become the FDA, and set about ousting homeopathy from the medical establishment. No research on homeopathic medicine was allowed to be published in any medical journal, which effectively silenced the homeopaths and prevented the public from being informed about the efficacy of homeopathic treatment. Many homeopathic hospitals were shut down, and homeopaths and all other alternative health practices were discredited.

My children were not vaccinated again after my eldest child became ill following vaccination injections at the age of three months, and again at six months. When I saw how feverish and puffy and distressed he became after those two injections, with eczema breakouts, it was clear to me that these vaccines, or innoculations, were causing more harm than good.

After each vaccination injection, his sleeping pattern became disrupted so that he only cat-napped for a wee while, and he would awaken with stomach pain which caused him to become very restless and to cry for hours. He had been a so-called 'good' baby before that first injection.

After the first injection at three months, it took around two or three months before his system had settled down again, by which time he was due for the second injection, and after which injection, the same scenario followed.

And so I endeavoured to seriously study homeopathy and natural medicine, so that we could treat the common illnesses ourselves, without having to go to the doctor and take unknown antibiotics or other drugs for the common childhood illnesses which happened to be doing the rounds.

Colour Therapy For Fever
Blue light left on in the bedroom at night, in conjunction with a homeopathic remedy, were effective in bringing down childhood fevers within a couple of hours. I always kept several blue light bulbs on hand, in case of sudden fevers and infections.

Vitamin Therapy For Childhood Diseases
I found Vitamin therapy to be effective for Measles, Mumps, Chickenpox, Croup and others. Vitamin C and Vitamin A, in higher than normal doses, are helpful in preventing or treating the severity of symptoms of the common childhood diseases. Vitamins C and A both quicken the healing process with measles, mumps or chickenpox.

These two vitamins can be taken before your child gets sick, when an outbreak of these childhood illnesses is about. They will do much to prevent or minimise the effects of the illnesses should your child succumb to these illnesses, which they most likely will do.

Vitamin C For Measles Mumps And Chickenpox
The best type is the form of calcium ascorbate, or Ester C, which is non-acidic. Either of these can be given safely in larger doses when treating an illness. Give every half an hour for around six doses.
As a preventative, an adult can take 1000 mg several times a day: between 4000 mg and 9000 mg of calcium ascorbate in doses of 1000 mg each. For a child around 7 to 12, half this dose: 500 mg of

calcium ascorbate, several times a day; more often, and in larger doses if treating a severe illness.

For children younger than 5, give just a quarter of a tablet, around 250 mg per dose.

The patient should drink plenty of water, or hot lemon drinks. Lemon drinks promote the good effect of the Vitamin C.

Vitamin A For Measles Mumps And Chickenpox

With Vitamin A you need to be careful with the dose, and not continue it too long, since it is accumulative. At the onset of the illness, you could use roughly twice the recommended amount for a child, but only for around three doses over 16 hours, by which time you should see an improvement. Then stop giving the Vitamin A for two days. Continue with the normal recommended dose after that.

Homeopathy And Childhood Diseases

Homeopathy works just as well, as a prophylactic, or as a means to minimise the severity of these diseases. You need to study the remedies a little, so that the best remedy is chosen.

Here are some remedies which have been recommended by well-known homeopath W.A. Dewey who wrote 'Practical Homeopathic Therapeutics' (1996). I used some of these remedies with great success in treating childhood illnesses.

Homeopathy For Measles Aconite: Great for the sudden onset of any illness. In measles use when there is fever and restlessness, can't stand the light, coryza and a croupy cough.

Arsen alb.: This is a prophylactic for many illnesses, including flu and measles. A wonderful remedy, both prophylactic and curative. It can be used in measles if the patient has deteriorated with diarrhoea, great weakness, delirium and restlessness.

Bryonia: This is a good chest remedy which can be helpful in measles in the second stage of the illness. It can help lung afflictions, especially if there is a dry cough, chest pain and overall aches and pain. It helps to bring out the rash.

Drosera: This is a favourite of mine. It is an excellent remedy for Whooping Cough and Croup in children and in adults. It is a prophylactic for whooping cough. Drosera caused a quick recovery in my young children on the many occasions when measles, mumps and chickenpox were raging in Auckland. It is a great measles remedy when there is whooping cough or croup.

Euphrasia: Use when there is profuse mucous discharge. Eyes are characteristically red and swollen and watery. Dry cough. Perhaps sore throat and hoarseness. Throbbing headache which lessens when the spots come out.

Gelsemium: Dewey considers this remedy very important in measles. For high fever with chilliness and croupy dry cough. Patient wants to be left alone. He says it is great for the second part of the illness when the spots appear, because gelsemium has a distinct effect on the skin.

Pulsatilla: W.A. Dewey recommends this remedy for the later stages of the disease. Usually there is little fever with Pulsatilla, but a lot of running nose and discharges. Mucous build up might cause earache, which is common with this remedy. The eyes might be gluey and sticky. A dry cough at night but better during the day. Mucous in the digestive system and diarrhoea with earache, a dry cough and little fever could indicate Pulsatilla.

Homeopathy For Mumps

Belladonna: This is an important homeopathic remedy for Mumps. Dewey rates it as number one.

Use at the onset of the illness, when the glands are swollen , red and hot. They hurt when pressed. Pains are usually worse on the right side, extending up to the ear, but not always.

Homeopathic Belladonna is also useful for the second stage of mumps, when headache and delirium may follow.

Mercurius: This is another highly recommended remedy for mumps.

Dewey refers to it in his book, 'Practical Homeopathic Therapeutics'. It has a great effect on the salivary glands, and it is often used in the second stage of mumps, when the fever has come down slightly, but with much salivation, smelly breath and sores coming out.

Pulsatilla: This is recommended by W.A. Dewey for both boys and girls, for glandular complications arising from mumps, such as orchitis, or mammary gland or ovarian problems. Symptoms for this remedy include a thickly coated tongue, dry mouth, and pain increasing in the evenings.

Rhus Tox: This can be used for left-sided mumps, when there are dark red or purplish swellings. Lachesis is another remedy for left-sided mumps.

With Rhus Tox, the limbs ache. The patient is very restless and symptoms worsen after dark.

Dr. Dewey indicates it for erysipelatous inflammation and typhoid conditions.

Dewey goes on to list some other more obscure but useful remedies for Mumps:

Pilocarpine muriate 3x for when the parotid gland is affected.

Conium for very hard swellings. Conium is well-known for its ability to soften and reduce tumours of any kind.

Clematis and Aurum for young males with orchitic complications.

Pulsatilla for metastases of ovaries in females.

Chickenpox Remedies

W.A. Dewey's book does not cover specifics for chicken pox.

I have listed those recommended for the disease which are listed in Miranda Castro's book 'The Complete Homeopathy Handbook', published by Macmillan London Limited, 1990.

Aconite: This is the first remedy to use, according to M. Castro. Others to consider are Ant. crud, Ant. tart., Belladonna, Mercurius, Pulsatilla, Rhus tox and Sulphur.

Rhus tox and Sulphur: Either of these can be used to relieve intense itching.

Antimon Tart: A good remedy for bringing out the rash.

Mercurius-s: Recommended for when the rash is suppurating and sore.

Chapter 17

Anti Cancer Homeopathic Remedies

Homeopathy Can Help Prevent Cancer

Homeopathy is a powerful medicine. It is an amazing science which rationalists cannot explain, as it works on the principle of 'like heals like', and on the principle of the 'minimum dose', the science of which escapes most people.

Actually, there are some treatments accepted in allopathic medicine which use the 'like to treat like' principle, but the use of microscopic doses of a substance to heal a condition, or prevent one occurring, is peculiar to homeopathy, and this is the thing which sceptics just cannot get their heads around.

But, homeopathy does work, and many medical doctors around the world have undergone study in homeopathic medicine in order to become proficient at prescribing homeopathic remedies for their patients.

Homeopathy is studied as a science and widely used in India: many developments in the proving of new remedies have come from studies done in India. Most of the literature on homeopathy is published in India.

Many doctors have found homeopathy to be invaluable as a preventative medicine, and in obtaining actual cures for many of their patients. Often, when allopathic medicine has failed to work in effecting a cure, homeopathy has brought people back to total health.

The Queen Mother was a great fan of homeopathic medicine. She lived beyond a hundred years. The Royal family have their own Royal Homeopath, which is, I think, a wonderful endorsement for homeopathic medicine.

The Homeopathic text entitled 'Indications of Miasm', by Dr. Harimohan Choudhury, (reprint 1999), gives detailed advice on the use of homeopathic medicine for cancer. Dr. Choudhury also has chapters in this book on the different miasms, and the treatments for the diseases which come under those categories.

Below are listed some of the homeopathic remedies which Dr. Choudhury suggests as anti-cancer remedies. I must point out, though, that unless you have knowledge and experience with the use of homeopathic medicine, it will be difficult to find the right remedy for one's own treatment. Just taking one 'out of the box' will probably not work. You do need to see an experienced homeopathic practitioner so that the correct remedy for your condition may be ascertained. It is important that the right remedy be chosen. Every remedy has different symptoms which correspond to a specific physical, mental and emotional conditions. The physical, mental, emotional, digestive and spiritual characteristics of the individual need to be assessed for every individual case, before considering the range of homeopathic remedies available.

It must be remembered that a homeopathic remedy just on its own is not enough to combat cancer. Appropriate treatment of any serious disease would include good nutrition, plenty of rest, and periods of fasting. With these prerequisites, the right homeopathic treatment could very well effect a cure, or at least make the patient more comfortable for the duration of his or her life.

Dr. Choudhury recommends fasting once a week for cancer patients; proper rest and recreation, which would include a period of thirty minutes rest daily after lunch; regular time for going to bed; regular pleasant walks each day; and the confidence and belief that you will be cured.

He recommends avoiding overuse of salt, sugar and fat, especially fatty meats. Not too much spicy food should be taken, and nor should meals be too large. All cosmetics which contain any chemicals should be avoided. And, of course, one should really ensure that one does not come into contact with insecticides, pesticides, or herbicides. In short, avoid contact with chemicals in the domestic environment, and avoid food which has any preservative or colouring or flavour added.

The A Grade Anti Cancer Homeopathics which Dr. Harimohan Choudhury lists are: Argentum. n., Arsenicum. alb., Arsenicum. iod., Asafoetida., Aurum. met., Aurum. mur. nat., Bismuth., Bromine., Calc. ars., Carb.ac., Carbo. an., Carcinosin, Card. m., Carb. sulph., Carb. veg., Chelidonium., Cholesterinum, Cinnamonium, Condu., Conium., Echinacea, Hoang-n., Hydrastis, Iodine, Iscador, which comes from mistletoe, , Kreosote, Lachesis, Lapis alb., Lycopodium, Mag. m., Medo, Mercurius. s., Nitric . acid, Ornithog., Phosphorus., Phytolacca., Rad. br., Scirrhinum., Sempervinum, Secale. c., Silicea, Stron. c., Syph., Tarentula Hisp., Thuja., Thapsi., Visc. alb., X-ray.

The B Grade Anti Cancer Homeopathics which Dr. Harimohan Choudhury recommends are: Aconite r., Alumn., Apis., Ambra, Anthrac, Ant. chlorid, Arg. m., Aster. Aur. ars., Aur. mur., Bufo., Cadmium., Calcarea. carb., Calc. s., China.., Cist. c., Cleam., Crot.h., fuligo lign., Galium., Geran. m., Graphites., Hamamelis., Ignatia., Iris. v., Kali c., Kali. ars., Kali. bi., Kali. iod., Kali. chl., Kali. cy., Kali. p., Kali. s., Morph., Murex, Muri ac., Merc, iod. fl., Mat.c., Mat. cacodylate., Nat. m., Plumbum. iod., Psorin., Rab.b., Rubi., Ruta., Scrofularia., Sepia, Spongia., Staphisagria., Sulphur., Zincum.

Many of these same remedies are recommended for the treatment of tumours in other texts. In the book 'Practical Homeopathic Therapeutics', by W.A. Dewey, (reprint 1996), we find a list of remedies which compares to that of Dr. Harimohan Choudhury's

above. The remedies which Dr. W.A. Dewey considers to be most important of these would seem to be the following:
Arsenicum, Calcarea fluor., Carbo an., Conium, and Hydrastis.
However, he also includes Baryta carb., Baryta iod., Bromine, Carbo veg., Carbolic acid, Cedron, Cicuta, Cundurango, Cuprum, Heda lava, Iodine, Kali sulph., Lapis alb., Morphine, Phosphorus, Phytolacca, Plumbum, Radium, Silicea, and Thuja.

Chapter 18

List Of Complementary Homeopathic Remedies And Sequences

What Sequence Of Homeopathic Remedies Work Best?

It is useful to know what homeopathic remedies work in harmony with each other. Some remedies complement each other, whilst other remedies may antidote the effect of a remedy already given. Remember not to drink coffee when you are using homeopathic remedies, since coffee is one of the main antidotes to homeopathy. It is also best to avoid perfumes, strong tea, garlic, alcohol, and strong spices whilst using the remedies.

Poisons such as fly spray, herbicides and other agricultural chemicals, should always be avoided by the person who is interested in protecting the health of the family. These poisons will also affect the efficacy of any homeopathic remedies you may be taking.

Usually, we hope, just one remedy will work to cure most complaints. I mainly used homeopathic Drosera for croup, or whooping cough, because my children responded well to this remedy. Aconite usually cures ailments which come on suddenly after being chilled or getting wet, and Belladonna will usually fix those high temperatures when the child has red, flushed cheeks.

But sometimes, when complications have arisen, or in other unusual cases–such as treating a young pup who suddenly was stricken down with the Parvo virus after I had agreed to foster him until we found him a home–it may be necessary to use a sequence of Homeopathic remedies to effect a final cure. In this case, I had to use a combination of remedies in order to rid the animal of the deadly Parvo virus, which took some beating. I kept feeding the poor wee thing with teaspoons of honey and water to keep it from being dehydrated.

Initial progress was made with Arsen alb., (or Mercurius) which brought down the temperature. This seemed not to be having any more good effect after a couple of days, so I followed with a day or two of Sulphur and Thuja, if I remember correctly. Even then, the final solution was to give the pup a dose of castor oil, which had the effect of immediately cleaning out the bowel, and the grateful puppy suddenly, and surprisingly, got up on its feet again, after having been at death's door for several days. Within a couple of weeks after its recovery, we found a wonderful home for this lucky wee chap.

Such was my happy experience in using homeopathy for dogs.

Complementary Homeopathic Remedies

The complementaries which have been found to be most effective for each given remedy are highlighted in the list which follows. Of course, you would choose the complementary remedy which most replicates the symptoms of your patient.

List Of Complementary Homeopathic Remedies And Sequences

This table is similar to that given by Harvey Farrington, M.D., who wrote 'Homeopathy and Homeopathic Prescribing'. This was reprinted in 2006 by B. Jain Publishers, India, and is available online. I have added information into this from Dr. J.H. Clarke's 'The Prescriber: How To Practice Homeopathy', which is also available from B. Jain Publishers, and from other textbooks, or from my own experience.

ACONITE is followed well by Arnica; Belladonna; Bryonia; Coffea; Mill; Phosphorous; Spongia; and Sulphur. It is related to Belladonna, Chamomilla, Coffea.

Dr John Renner used Aconite 3x and Bryonia 3x, given both together at the same time, every 30 minutes during childbirth. He brought thousands of babies into the world using this combination. (Ullman 1988)

ACTEA SPICATA is complementary to Caul; Colo.; Sabi.; Stict.; Vio-o. (Phatack, 1977) Useful for swollen, painful joints, especially of wrist, fingers or ankles. Old people sensitive to cold. Change in weather often brings on symptoms. Sometimes shortness of breath with cold weather. A bluish tinge to the sight.

ADONIS VERNALIS Phatack says this is a great non-cumulative heart remedy, especially in cases where heart is weakened following rheumatism, influenze, nephritis, or due to fatty degeneration. Can help regulate the pulse and strengthen muscles of the heart, help urine flow and improve conditions such as arrrhythmia, cardiac dropsy, hydrothorax, ascites, anasarca. Phatack claims it for 'Compensatory hypertrophy of heart in cardiac stenosis and mitral regurgitation.' His dose is 5-10 drops of the homeopathic tincture. It is related to Bufo. and can be compared with Conval; Digitalis; Strop.

ALOES is followed well by Sulphur.

ALUMINA is followed well by Bryonia; Ferr.m. Alumina is complementary to Bryonia and related to both Bryonia and Plumbum. Useful for female complaints, especially gynoecological.

ANT. CRUD. is followed well by Squill.

ANTIMON TART is followed well by Baryta carbonica; Ipecacuanha.

APIS is followed well by Arnica; Baryta carbonica; Merc. cy; Nat. mur; Pulsatilla.
One popular commercial combination is Apis, Belladonna and Phytolacca.
Apis mellifica - Should not be given after Rhus tox. Apis is complementary to Nat mur. (T.S. Iyer p.364)

ARGENTUM NITR. is followed well by Kali c; Nat. mur.

ARNICA is followed well by Aconite; Calc. carb; Natr. sulph; Psor; Rhus tox; Sul. ac.
Some common and effective Arnica combinations are:
Arnica, Asafoetida, and Pulsatilla.
Aconite, Mercurius, and Arnica.
Arnica, Asafoetida, and Rhus Tox.
Arnica, Aconite,and Rhus Tox.
Arnica, Mercurius, and Rhus Tox.
Arnica, Ipecac., and Aconite.
Pulsatilla, Arnica, and Lycopodium.

ARSENICUM ALB. is a much used remedy. It is followed well by Allium sativum; Carbo veg; Lachesis; Natr. sul; Phos.; Pulsatilla; Sulphur; Thuja.
Harvey Farrington M.D. often uses Arsenicum followed by Belladonna.
Arsenicum alb. is also followed well by: Nux vomica; Iodine; Rhus tox.; (skin diseases) Sulphur. He lists as complementaries to Arsen alb.: Carbo veg; Phosphorus; Thuja; Secale.
Arsen alb. follows well AFTER: Aconite; Agaricus; Arnica; Belladonna; Chamomilla; China; Ipecac; Lachesis; Veratrum alb. (Farrington).
Arsen alb. antidotes: Carbo veg; China; Ferrum met.; Graphites; Hepar sulph; Iodine; Ipecac; Nux vom; Mercurius; Phosphorus; Sambucus; Tabacum; Veratrum alb.
Arsen alb. is an antidote for lead poisoning, as well as for various types of food poisoning.
Arsen alb. is antidoted by the following remedies: Camphor; China; Ferrum met; Graphites; Hepar sulph; Iodine; Ipecac; Nux vom; Sambusux; Tabacum; Veratrum alb.
Arsen alb is used together in a commercial preparation with Gelsemium and Eupatorium Perf. I find

this combination very good for shingles and eczema when dairy milk is excluded from the diet.

ARUM TRI is followed well by Nitric acid.

ASAFOETIDA is followed well by Causticum; Pulsatilla. The sequence of Asafoetida, China, Mercurius, and Pulsatilla is a recommended one.
Arnica can be followed by Asafoetida and then Rhus Tox.
One sequence which is frequently used is Asafoetida, Lycopodium, Pulsatilla.
Asafoetida will antidote some remedies, if given after them: It antidotes Causticum, Camphor, China, Mercurius, Pulsatilla and Valerian.

BARYTA CARB is followed well by Antimon tart. It is useful to use either before or after Hepar sulph, Psorinum, Sulphur, and Tub. Dr Adolph Von Lippe says that using Psorinum after Baryta carb can 'eradicate the constitutional tendency to quinsy'.

BELLADONNA is followed well by Bor; Calc. carb; Hepar sulph; Mercurius; Nat. mur.

BRYONIA is followed well by Abro; Alum; Kali c; Lycopodium; Rhus tox.; Sepia; Sulphur.
Dr Adolph Von Lippe recommends Phytolacca to follow, if Bryonia and Rhus tox do not have effect.

CALCAREA CARB. is followed well by Bar. c; Lycopodium; Silica.

CALCAREA FLUOR. is followed well by Rhus tox.

CALCAREA PHOS. is followed well by Ruta; Sulphur; Zinc.

CANTHARIS is followed well by Apis.

CAPSICUM is followed well by Nat. mur.

CARBO AN. is followed well by Calc. phos.

CARBO VEG. is followed well by Arsen alb; China; Kali c.; Lachesis; Phosphorous. Dr J. N. Singhal lists Kali carb and Drosera as complementary to Carbo veg. He compares Carbo veg to Carboneum; Lycopodium; Veratrum album; Carbolic acid.

Singhal complements Carbo veg. with Kali carb. for chest troubles. For haemorrhage and dysepsia, he complements Carbo veg. with China.

Carbo veg. is commonly used for collapsed states and chronic conditions, (Boericke) in 30th potency or higher. Dr Banerjee uses the 6th potency for chronic cases with wind in the upper part of stomach, or Lycopodium if wind is in the abdomen. Dr Bhardwaj uses high potencies, eg C.M., for collapsed states. Dr Singhal says that Carbo veg. can help save lives after severe illness such as typhoid, cholera, pneumonia, when the vital force is extremely low.

Carbo veg. for stomach complaints when Nux vom. fails to act, (Farrington), for stopping internal bleeding, (followed by China), whooping cough, and asthmatic attacks in elderly, when there is much perspiration and heat, especially on forehead. Note: Veratrum alb. is another important remedy for near collapse, but with Veratrum album, the sweat is cold. Hoarseness often goes with Carbo veg..

CAUSTICUM Potassium hydrate or Caustic potash. Acts on nerves, muscles, bladder. It is followed well by Carbo. veg; Graphites; Lachesis; Petros.; Sepia; Stan.; Staph. Related to Gel.; Kali-bi.; Pho.;

Rhus tox.; Sepea. Dr Phatak recommends Causticum for retention of urine after an operation. For children slow to walk and talk. Chewing difficult. Effects of lead poisoning. Anxious and sad. Feels guilty as if responsible for some crime. Negative outlook. Spoonerisms in speech, jumbling up order of words or letters. Warts. Restless legs at night. Rheumatic pains, cramps in legs, taught tendons, stiff joints, weak ankles, difficulty walking.

CEANOTHUS A great spleen remedy. Complementary to Nat. mur. and related to China. For enlarged liver or spleen, and useful for leukemia. Pain on left side under rib cage. Better for lying on right side.

CEPA is followed well by Phos.; Pulsatilla; Sarsaparilla; Thuja.

CHAMOMILLA is followed well by Belladonna; Calc. carb.; Mag. c.; Sanic.

CHELIDONIUM is followed well by Lycopodium or Merc.d.; or follow Lycopodium with Chelidonium if the first does not work. Related remedies: Bryonia; Kali-bi.; Mercurius; Opium. Chelidonium is a great liver remedy, acting more on the right side. Characteristic to Chelidonium is a yellow tinge to the complexion and upset stomach, which indicates liver malfunction, or jaundice. Affects the right lower lung and right side of abdomen. Right-sided pain. Better for lying on stomach. Feels anxious as if guilty of a crime. Worse for change of weather, coughing, motion and at 4.pm and 4.am.

CHINA is followed well by Arsen alb.; Cal. p.; Carbo veg.; Ferr.; Kali c.;

CINA is followed well by Calc. c.; Drosera; Sulphur.

COCCULUS is followed well by Petr.

COFFEA is followed well by Aconite.

COLCHICUM is followed well by Arsen alb.; Spigelia.

COLOCYNTHUS is followed well by Causticum; Mercurius; Staphisagria.

CONIUM is followed well by Phosphorus; Silica.

CROTALUS HORRIDUS is a homeopathic remedy derived from the snake of the same name. Like Lachesis, another snake remedy, it is a left-sided remedy which affects the nervous system and the heart, and shares many of the same symptoms, except it is worse for cold air. Its complementary is Lycopus.
Related remedies to Crotalus are: The Ophedia; Arsen alb.; Camphor; Carbo veg.; Lachesis; Laur.; Sul. ac.; Tarentula cub.

CUPRUM is followed well by Arsen alb.; Calc. carb.; Iodum.

DROSERA is followed well by Carbo. veg.; Nux vomica; Sulphur.

DULCAMARA is followed well by Alum.; Baryta carb.; Nat. sulph.

EUPATORIUM PERF is followed well by Nat mur and Sepia

FERRUM is followed well by Alumina; Arsen alb.; China; Hamamelis.

FERRUM PHOS. is followed well by Nat. mur.

FLUORIC ACID is followed well by Silica.

GELSEMIUM is followed well by Argent. nit.; Sepia.
The combination of Gelsemium, Hydrastis and Calendula, given 3x per day, 3 drops of each, was given by a Dr. Gerald Gibb, of Auckland, for a friend of mine who had severe agricultural poisoning, which included Dieldrin, RoundUp, and other chemicals. This treatment was followed for many months, and eventually proved effective in clearing the body of the poisons which were making her so sick.

GLONOIN is followed well by Belladonna.

GRAPHITES is followed well by Arsen alb.; Causticum; Ferr. met.; Hepar sulphuris; Lycopodium; Sulphur.

HAMAMELIS is followed well by Ferr. met.; Fluoricum Acidum.

HELLEBORUS is followed well by Zinc.

HEPAR SULPHURIS is followed well by Iodum; Silica.

IGNATIA is followed well by Nat. mur.; Phos. acidum; Pulsatilla; Sepia.

IODINE is followed well by Badiag.; Lycopodium; Silica.

IPECACUANHA is followed well by Arsen alb.; Cuprum metallicum.

KALI BICHROMICUM is followed well by Arsen alb.; Phosphorus ; Psorinum.

KALI CARBONICUM is followed well by Arsenicum iodatum; Carbo veg.; Nitric acid; Phosphorus.

KALI MUR is followed well by Calcarea sulphurica.

KALMIA is followed well by Benzoicum acidum; Spigelia.

KREOSOTE is followed well by Sulphur.

LACHESIS is chiefly a left-sided remedy which is followed well by Arsen alb.; Calcarea carbonicum; Carbo veg.; Hepar sulph; Lycopodium; Mitric acidum; Phosphorus; Zinc iodide.
Dr. Farrington lists the related remedies of Lachesis as: Arsen alb.; Belladonna; Carbo veg.; Causticum; Conium; Hepar sulph.; Lycopodium; Mercurius; Nitric acid; Sepia; Tarent. cub.; Tarent. hisp.; Zinc; and the Ophidia.
Lycopodium, Phosphorus, Zinc and Iodine are particularly complementary to Lachesis.

LACTIC ACID is followed well by Psorinum.

LEDUM is followed well ty China; Sepia. Ledum is reputed to be a prophylactic for tetanus.

LYCOPODIUM is followed well by Calcarea carbonica; Iodum; Kali c.; Lachesis; Phosphorus; Pulsatilla; Sulphur.

MAGNESIUM C is followed well by Chamomilla.

MARUM VERUM is followed well by Calcarea carbonica.

MERCURIUS is followed well by Aurum metallicum; Badiag.; Belladonna; Hepar sulphuris; Sepia; Sulphur.

Mercurius also follows well after Belladonna; Hepar sulphuris; Lachesis or Sulphur, but should Sulphur should never be given after Silicea according to T.S. Iyer.

NAJA is not such a common remedy, but it has its uses. It is related to Lachesis: Both are snake remedies which affect the nervous system and the heart. Naja, according to Harvey Farrington, is often more useful than Lachesis for heart affections such as angina pectoris with pains going to shoulder and neck; for heart palpitations brought on by stress; frontal headaches accompanied by pains in spine and palpitations; myocarditis with stitching pains due to stress; uncomplicated cardiac hypertrophy in young people.

Naja's related remedies: Arsen alb.; Cactus; Carbo veg.; Camphor; Cimic.; Tab.; Lachesis; Laur.; the Ophidia.

NATRUM CARBONICA is followed well by Sepia.

NATRUM MUR is followed well by Apis; Arg. nit.; Ignatia; Sepia.

NATRUM SULPH. is followed well by Arsen alb.; Thuja.

NITRIC ACID is followed well by Arsen alb.; Arum t.; Calad.; Calc. carbonica; Lycopodium; Thuja.

NUX MOSCHATA is followed well by Calcarea carbonica; Lycopodium.

NUX VOMICA is followed well by Bryonia; Chamomilla; Conium; Kali carbonica; Phosphorus; Pulsatilla; Sepia; Sulphur.

OPIUM is followed well by Alumina; Baryta carbonica; Bryonia; Phosphorus; Plumbum.

PALLADIUM is followed well by Platina.

PETROLEUM is followed well by Sepia.

PHOSPHORIC ACID is followed well by China.

PHOSPHORUS is followed well by Arsen alb.; Calcarea carbonica; Cepa; Kali carbonica; Lycopodium; Sanguinaria canadensis; Sepia; Silica; Sulphur.

PHYTOLACCA is complemented by Silica. It is antidoted by Belladonna and Mezerium. Mercurius is incompatible with Phytolacca. Phytolacca is a great gland remedy, and is especially known for its action on the breast and its mammary glands. Can be used for reducing breast lumps. Its action is similar to Bryonia and Rhus tox: Phytolacca will often produce a cure when these two remedies fail to act.

I have found that, in combination with non-acidic Vitamin C, 10,000 mg a day thereabouts, for as long as needed and dose depending on the severity of the condition, Phytolacca taken daily for three weeks at a time, then a break, combined with Bryonia and weekly dose of Arsen alb has cured the type of breast lump which occurs after exposure to toxic herbicides such as glyphosate in RoundUp.

PLUMBUM is followed well by Rhus toxicodendron.

PODOPHYLLUM is followed well by Calcarea carbonica; Nat mur.; Sulphur.

PSORINUM is followed well by Sepia; Sulphur; Tuberc.

PULSATILLA is followed well by Arsen alb.; Bryonia; Kali bich.; Kali sulph.; Lycopodium; Sepia; Silica; Stannum; Sulphur; Sulph. acid; Zinc. Harvey Farrington M.D. uses the combination Pulsatilla; Arnica; Lycopodium to good effect.

RHEUM is followed well by Magnesia carbonica.

RHUS TOXICODENDRON is followed well by Bryonia; Calcarea carbonica; Causticum; Lycopodium; Medorrhinum; Phosphorus; Phytolacca; Pulsatilla; Sulphur.

RUTA is followed well by Calcarea phos.

SABADILLA is followed well by Sepia.

SABINA is followed well by Thuja.

SANGUINARIA is followed well by Antimon tart.; Phosphorus.

SARSAPARILLA is followed well by Mercurius; Sepia.

SECALE is followed well by Arsen alb.; Thuja.

SEPIA is followed well by Nat. mur.; Phosphorus; Psorinum; Pulsatilla; Sulphur.

SILICA is followed well by Fluoricum acidum; Hepar sulphuris; Lycopodium; Phosphorus; Thuja.

SPIGELIA is followed well by Spongia.

SPONGIA is followed well by Hepar sulphuris

SQUILLA is followed well by Antimonium crudum.

STANNUM is followed well by Pulsatilla.

STAPHYSAGRIA is followed well by Causticum; Colocynthis.

SULPHUR is followed well by Aconite; Aloe; Arsenicum album; Badiaga; Belladonna; Calcarea carbonica; Mercurius; Pulsatilla; Psorinum; Pyrogen (also called Sepsin); Rhus toxicodendron; Sepia; Sulphuricum iodide.
Aloe and Psorinum are complementary to Sulphur, and can be used concurrently with Sulphur.

Iyer says to use Sulphur after Aconite - useful sometimes in cases of pneumonia or other acute disease. Iyer also recommends the following sequences: Sulphur, Calcarea, Lycopodium, or Sulphur, Sarsparilla, Sepia.

SULPHURIC ACID is followed well by Pulsatilla.

THUJA is followed well by Mercurius; Nat. mur; Nitric acid; Pulsatilla; Sabina; Silica; Sulphur.

TUBERCULINUM is followed well by Calcarea carbonica; Kali sulph.; Sepia.

VERATRUM ALBUM is followed well by Arsenicum album; Carbo veg.: (Farrington) These three remedies are the top three listed by Hahnemann for near collapse of the body's functions, when diseases such as cholera, typhoid, asthma, bronchitis, or pneumonia have weakened the body so much that death might seem imminent. Veratrum album is called for when the vital organs are about to give up, with an overall cold sweat. Carbo veg. usually has a hot perspiration on the forehead, but rest of body may be cold and blue. (Dr J.N. Singhal)

ZINCUM is followed well by Pulsatilla; Sepia; Sulphur.

Note: Even holding the appropriate remedy, or thinking about it, can have the desired effect, I find. The following excerpt from a report to the New Zealand Director-General of Health ('Task Force on Chronic Agricultural Chemical Poisoning Notifications', 1986) confirms that holding a remedy can effect a change in a patient:
Dr. Voll writes 'In 1954 I gave a demonstration of electroacupuncture diagnosis to a small group of friends in Germany. I diagnosed one colleague as having chronic prostatitis and advised him to take Homeopathic preparation called Echinaceae 4X.
He replied that he had this medication in his office and went to get it. When he returned with the bottle of Echinaceae in his hand, I tested the prostate measurement point again and made the discovery that the point reading which was previously up to 90, had decreased to 64 which was an enormous improvement of the prostate value.
I had the colleague put the bottle aside and the previous measurement value returned. After holding the medication in his hand the measurement value went down to 64 again and this pattern repeated itself as often as desired. This procedure could therefore be reproduced.'

Chapter 19

Complete List Of Gluten-Free Foods For People With Wheat Sensitivity

Personally, I believe that glyphosate in the herbicide 'RoundUp', and in so-called 'RoundUp-Ready' crops which are resistant to glyphosate, but nevertheless absorb the poison, is causing widespread ill health. Our bodies now contain 500 times more glyphosate than they did in 1994, when genetically modified crops were developed to withstand any amount of the herbicide glyphosate.

If you have problems with your digestion, with diarrhea or constipation, or both these conditions, then you could be sensitive not only to the gluten found in wheat, rye flour and barley, but more to glyphosate, which is high in these grain crops, and is also found in dairy products too. Try to use organic products as much as possible, to reduce the intake of glyphosate and other agricultural chemicals.

Note: Do see a health practitioner if you have any problems with digestion or overall health.

You might have been diagnosed with coeliac disease: Both the coeliac condition and allergy or sensitivity to gluten respond well to wheat products, barley and rye being eliminated from the diet. If your problem is coeliac disease, then you will be best to avoid dairy products and sugar as well, at least until your condition improves.   But if your problem is specifically gluten sensitivity, then you will find your condition improves, radically and dramatically, simply by leaving out wheat, rye, barley, and all foods which may contain gluten.

It is reasonable to suspect that the gluten in wheat and other food items might be the problem if you have diarrhea, or constipation, irritable bowel syndrome, colitis, a distended stomach, stomach cramps or discomfort after eating a meal, sinus trouble, skin problems, depression, candida and symptoms of malnutrition due to your food not being processed properly, with accompanying listlessness and a lack of motivation to tackle important tasks.

Of course there are other conditions which can cause the above symptoms, so if you have any of these symptoms, then it is best to see a health professional to get a proper medical diagnosis.

I find that my system tolerates rye bread well when I consume freshly made vegetable and apple juices each day, whilst supplementing the diet with a small teaspoon of Kruschen Salts every second morning, dissolved in half a cup of hot water and then cooled before drinking. Kruschen Salts are high in magnesium, which helps reduce acidity, and seems to improve my tolerance to some grains, rye being more tolerable than wheat.

Meanwhile, you might try a gluten-free diet using suggestions from the following complete list of gluten-free foods to see whether your condition improves.

Doing without gluten in your cooking and your daily diet is actually an easy thing. Take heart, because you can survive very well without products like wheat flour, rye and barley. You can also improve your nutrition enormously by using other organic foods instead of the daily bread and wheat-laden foods to which we are accustomed.

We find the ubiquitous wheat with its problematic gluten in many commercially produced foods such as sausages, sausage meat, baked beans, textured vegetable protein, sauces, soups, and corn flakes. Make sure you avoid all such products and use only the foods from the complete list of gluten-free foods, unless, of course, the product indicates specifically that it is gluten free.

It is far better to make all your meals from scratch, at home, using raw ingredients you can be sure are gluten free. Do this rather than buying any commercially made preparations or meals. If you do have a sensitivity to gluten, as yet undiagnosed, then you will find your health improving dramatically in a matter of weeks by using the recommended substitutes for wheat which are listed below.

Generally speaking, rice is the king of grains, best used to replace wheat and rye and barley. Rice is totally gluten free which is surprising since it has what we call a 'glutinous' make-up once it is cooked in plenty of water.
Use rice every day – at every meal if you wish.

Rice can replace those breakfast cereals which contain wheat. It can accompany a meal of protein such as fish, meat or chicken and leafy green vegetables, or it can accompany a vegetarian salad with nuts, seeds, almonds and avocado.

Rice, when made into flour can be used alone or in combination with other gluten-free grains in baking and makes the most delicious and nutritious cookies and desserts. These treats should be used only occasionally for most people.

For people with multiple sensitivities, candida or hyperglycaemia, sweet foods of any kind – along with dairy foods – are best left out until the condition improves. Butter is usually okay, though, as is ghee, a product made from butter. You can experiment with butter and ghee to see if they do suit you.

Brown rice, of course, is the most nutritious and the best type for the digestion, as the vitamins and fibre in the outer part of the rice are still intact. But white rice ground into flour is a good substitute for white wheat flour, to use in baking biscuits and cakes and bread.

Baking Gluten Free: Our complete list of gluten-free foods for people with wheat sensitivity will begin with the flours and grains which can substitute wheat and rye in your cooking. A mixture of chickpea flour, soy, rice and corn flours is generally a good mix to use in baking cookies and cakes, or to use for thickening stews and gravies.

Tapioca and arrowroot are also great gluten-free flours to help your baking rise. These flours do not contain any gluten and are therefore safe for people with gluten intolerance. Use rice flour for about half the measure of flour needed, and make up the rest of the quantity stated in the recipe with some soy and corn flours with a bit of tapioca or arrowroot flours added for lightness in baking.

Wheat-Free Baking Substitutes: Gluten-Free Flours and Grains
 Arrowroot Flour
 Buckwheat Groats and Flour
I have an idea that buckwheat may contain a type of gluten similar to that found in oats. This could be okay for most people, but be cautious with your use of buckwheat if you are very sensitive to gluten.

Chickpeas and chickpea or besan flour are safe, as is cornmeal - groats or finely milled yellow cornmeal.
Note about Cornflakes: Cornflakes are dubious, as some brands have malt added to them. Malt contains gluten. You really can't go wrong if you stick to the real yellow groats, or fine yellow cornmeal.

Ground millet is an especially nourishing breakfast cereal. Made into a porridge, it is good for people with delicate digestion, and the very young, as well as for those who have an intolerance to gluten.
Oats are not totally gluten free. They contain a

different type of gluten to wheat and rye, and this is a very small amount compared to that found in wheat or rye. Many people who are sensitive to gluten find they can tolerate small amounts of oats daily – half a cup in a porridge, or in cookies, is generally an acceptable amount.

However, in extreme cases of sensitivity to gluten, oats might best be left out, and millet porridge, or rice, used instead.

Pea Flour or chickpea flour

Potato Flour

Rice and Rice Flour

Soybeans and Soy Flour

Tapioca and Tapioca Flour

A Note on Milk

Dairy milk is gluten free. However, if you also wish to avoid dairy products, then you could choose from the following milks, which are also gluten free.

Almond Milk

Cashew Nut Milk

Coconut Milk

Rice Milk

Sesame Seed Milk

Sunflower Seed Milk

Soy Milk

Note: Check the product packaging on Soy Milk. Some brands may contain wheat products. Make sure you buy a brand whose labelling you can trust.

Gluten-Free Fruits and Vegetables

All root vegetables, and all leafy green vegetables are gluten free with the exception of the Jerusalem Artichoke, which has a small amount of a gluten type substance in its tuber.

Fruits are also gluten free. These foods are also better nutritionally for you than eating wheat flour bread, pastries and other wheat-based products, even if you are not gluten sensitive. This is because they provide good quality fibre and roughage to the bowel. Fibre encourages the growth of helpful organisms in the intestines, and acts as a natural cleanser. Fibre is just the thing to keep you healthy.

Vegetables and fruits also contain large amounts of vitamins and minerals which are not so abundant in cooked wheat flour. Vitamin C is high in all fruit and vegetables, especially when eaten raw. Where possible make fresh salads rather than cooking vegetables. Or eat a piece of fresh fruit as a snack. Of course, if you have hyperglycaemia as well as an intolerance to wheat and rye, then you will need to be careful with sweet fruits until your health has recovered.

Alfalfa Sprouts
 Apples
Apricots
Artichoke (Globe Artichoke, not the Jerusalem artichoke. The Jerusalem artichoke contains a type of gluten, as well as inulin.)
Asparagus
Aubergine or eggplant
Avocado
Bananas
Beetroot
Bilberries
Blackberries
Blackcurrants
Blueberries
Broad beans – dried or freshly picked.
Broccoli
Brussels Sprouts
Cabbage
Canteloup
Capers
Capsicum
Carrot
Cauliflower

Celery
Cherimoya
Cherries
Chick Pea Sprouts
Chinese Cabbage-Bok Choy, Chi Hi Li.
Chives
Coconut
Comfrey
Coriander
Corn
Cranberries
Cucumber
Cumin seed
Currants
Dates
Figs
Garlic
Ginger
Gooseberries
Grapes
Green Beans
Green Peppers
Kale
Kiwifruit
Kohlrabi
Kumara
Leeks
Lemons
Lettuce
Lima beans
Lychees
Mango
Melons – Watermelon and Rock Melon.
Mung Bean Sprouts (cooked Mung Beans are also gluten free.)
Mushrooms
Nectarines
Olives

Onions – all types of onions are gluten free.
Oranges (although many people cannot digest oranges so well.)
Parsnips
Passion Fruit
Paw Paw
Peaches
Peanuts (actually a legume.)
Peas
Peppers – red and green. Also chili peppers.
Persimmon
Pineapple
Plums
Pomegranate
Potato (and Potato flour for baking.)
Pumpkin
Raisins
Raspberries
Red Peppers
Rhubarb
Rocket
Salsify
Silver Beet
Spinach
Sugar Cane
Sugar Cane and Sugar Cane products such as molasses, treacle, golden syrup, and brown and white sugar are gluten free. Brown sugar and molasses are best, of course, as these contain chromium, zinc and other minerals and vitamins which are absent in white sugar. Unadulterated Honey is also gluten free. Maple Syrup is gluten free.
Sultanas
Swede
Sweet Potato (kumara)
Squash
Tamarillos
Taro
Tomatoes

Turmeric
Turnips
Yams

Fruit Juices
All fruit juices are gluten free. However, these should be taken in moderation, especially if your bowels are not yet operating normally. Sometimes citrus fruit juices are added to fruit-juice mixes – citrus fruits can be problematic for some people. In extreme cases, it might be best to avoid fruit juices until health is restored. Some people find a grape juice fast, or an apple juice fast to be helpful in the beginning of a treatment: best to get some professional advice on this before you attempt a juice fast, though.

Gluten-Free Protein Foods
You can eat any of the following gluten-free foods: Almonds, Cashews, Walnuts, Avocado, Fish, Meat, Tempeh, Tofu, Eggs, Nuts, Pumpkin Seeds, Sunflower Seeds, Sesame Seeds.

All Dairy Products – butter, cream, cheese, milk – are gluten free. However, some people might be best to leave dairy foods alone until they have recovered. Butter is generally tolerated by most people, even if they have sensitivities to milk and cheese. Butter is an ideal cooking fat, as it does not make the toxins which most oils do when heated.

All natural protein foods are gluten free. This means you can eat any fish or shellfish, all meats, beef, chicken, lamb, and eggs. Of course, you will try to choose free-range products. Tofu, a soy bean curd, is a very good protein-rich food, ideal for people on strict vegetarian diets. These protein foods are safe:
Beef
Lamb
Mutton
Tofu
Eggs

Fish – all shellfish, cod, eel, herrings, lemon fish, mackerel, mullet, mussels, oysters, salmon, sardines, snapper, tarakihi, tuna.

Protein-Rich Milks
The following milks are all gluten free.
Almond milk
Camel's milk
Coconut milk
Cow's milk
Goat's milk
Nut milk – made from cashews, hazelnuts, brazil nuts or walnuts.
Rice milk
Soy milk

Nuts, Pulses and Seeds
All nuts, pulses and seeds listed here are gluten free.
 Alfalfa – cooked, sprouted, or made into a tea.
 Almonds
 Black eyed beans or peas
 Broad beans – dried or fresh from the vine.
 Cashews
 Chickpeas – cooked, or sprouted, or used as a flour.
 Hazelnuts
 Lima beans
 Macadamia nuts
 Mung beans (cooked or sprouted.)
 Peanuts
Peas and pea flour
 Pumpkin seeds
 Red Kidney beans
 Soy beans
 Sunflower Seeds
 Tiger beans
Vegetable Oils
All vegetable oils are gluten free, and most are rich sources of Vitamin E and other goodies.

Easy, Organic Crock-Pot Bread
(Do not use if gluten sensitive)
Here is my easy recipe for making organic, yeast free bread, which may be tolerated by some people who usually find wheat or rye bread indigestible.

My system objects to commercial bread if I indulge over several days, whereas I find that this home made bread is easier to digest.

It reduces glyphosate intake by using organic flours, is yeast-free, and no extra gluten is added, which is a problem with commercial breads. It may be the answer for some people's allergies to yeast and various grains and gluten. (Ask doctor before trying)

This bread is made in a crock-pot or slow cooker.

2 medium cups of organic wholemeal wheat flour
2 medium cups of organic white flour (if using self-raising flours, then omit the baking powder)
1 cup of besan flour, or pea flour
1/2 cup dessicated coconut
1/2 cup ground linseed or ground sesame seeds
3 tablespoons olive oil
1 egg. 2 tsps salt. 3 teaspoons baking powder
2 cups cold water: Boil another 1/2 cup water, and mix in 1 teaspoon baking soda.

Mix up the flours with baking powder and other dry ingredients. Make a well at the centre of the flour and add the beaten egg, oil, water, and the baking soda water.

Mix as for bread and fold in the flour carefully. Do not stir too much. Put out onto a floured bench and knead for a few minutes, adding a little more flour or water if necessary, to create a nice, smooth dough.

Grease the inside and bottom of a 4-5 litre size crock-pot or slow cooker. Put in the dough, put on the lid and cook on high for exactly 2 hours. Cool on a wire tray. Keep in the fridge and use within 5 days. Eat with salad.

Chapter 20

Candida Albicans: Why It Happens, And How To Fix It

Yeast infections from Candida overgrowth: The candida albicans organism is one which occurs naturally in the digestive system. The balance of different bowel organisms sometimes becomes unstable though, and this can cause a wide range of distressing conditions.

The condition of candida overgrowth can include some or all of the following symptoms: memory loss, dizziness, recurring ear infection, ringing in the ears, weakness of the limbs, shingles, swollen glands, weakness of the lungs with recurring colds, blurred or cloudy vision, yeast infection, constipation or stools which are too loose, eczema, psoriasis, migraines, sleeplessness, restlessness, arthritic pain and depression.

Overgrowth of candida albicans happens when one's immune system becomes weakened. This can sometimes happen if the person has been traumatised by some event, but very often the cause of candida albicans becoming a problem is because of auto-intoxication resulting from a bad diet. This is usually a diet deficient in green vegetables and which contains too much processed and preserved food. This causes toxins to build up in the intestines which provides a hospitable environment for candida to breed.

Candida outbreaks can also strike when one is suddenly exposed to environmental factors such as radiation, or chemicals which are hazardous to the health, like farm herbicides and insecticides. Domestic poisons like fly spray, rat poison and cockroach killer can cause candida to flourish.

Even using products like bleach too frequently, or bath and shower cleaners, can cause an immediate imbalance in the bowel flora.

This is because the bleach is absorbed into the skin,

fumes get absorbed through the lungs, and from those organs the poison goes straight into the blood. It kills the useful organisms in the intestines in a similar way that chemicals such as glyphosate in RoundUp does.

If bleach fumes are taken into the mouth, the quality of your saliva is changed immediately, making it excessively alkaline. This affects digestion and encourages candida infection.

Heavy metal poisoning such as mercury or lead poisoning, and asbestos poisoning can leave the immune system severely weakened so that candida albicans can take control.

Candida infection can occur if one is exposed over a period of time to radiation such as that from cellphones, or electricity transformers and high tension electricity wires which are too close in proximity for the body to be able to function normally. Radiation, which will lower your immunity also kills off the beneficial bacteria in the bowel just as quickly as farm and domestic poisons do.

A diet too high in sugar will cause candida: even if the diet favours sweet fruit over eating green vegetables, then candida can result because of excessive sugar intake. Wheat flour is problematic because it is absorbed as sugar too quickly into the bloodstream. Eating too many yeast products can cause candida, especially if the diet is lacking green vegetables, oils, and protein. Foods containing yeast, especially bread, should be avoided.

Generally, if the the body is cleared of toxins, then candida should not be a problem. But sometimes it can take a long time to rebuild the immune system after it has been shaken, especially if the body has been exposed to prolonged periods of damaging environmental conditions.

Natural Remedies To Rid The Body Of Candida Without Antibiotics

Of course, you do need to consult with your doctor or naturopath or homeopath or ayurvedic practitioner before using any of these remedies. And you would generally use only one of the following methods, depending on what your health practitioner suggests.

And after trying a 'quick fix' to eliminate candida, you need to still take care with your diet and avoid yeasts, alcohol, sugar, milk products and wheat as much as possible.

Vaccinations and antibiotics can also cause candida infections. Even flu jabs can weaken your immune system by interfering with the natural balance of organisms in the intestines.

I have found some natural remedies which will tackle the onslaught of a sudden candida infection. They can reduce the distressing symptoms of candida very effectively.

These remedies are epsom salts, castor oil, calcium ascorbate, and enemas. Aspirin, baking soda, garlic, and the kawakawa leaf from the plant which is indigenous to New Zealand, are also helpful, but the first three mentioned are very quick to act, especially in conjunction with an enema. Of course, there are many other remedies, such as homeopathic thuja-echinacea, and herbs such as taheebo, or pau d'arco, but I will talk here about the remedies which are easy to procure in New Zealand, and inexpensive as well – Epsom Salts, Castor Oil, and Calcium Ascorbate.

1) A Candida Quick Fix Using Epsom Salts

This is very easy to do. It works by cleansing the effete matter out of the intestines and other organs. Rubbish hanging about in the body's digestive process is a great breeding ground for candida. Epsom salts also have an alkaline effect on the body and its digestive process; making the body alkaline through taking epsom salts for a few days stops the candida albicans from proliferating. Thus epsom salts is helpful in normalising and balancing the bowel flora again.

Dose for Epsom Salts as a quick fix for Candida:

Note: If you have heart problems, or are unwell from any other disease, then you should not try this remedy. Seek advice from your doctor.

If you are normally quite healthy then an adult can take a dose, first thing in the morning or last thing at night, of two teaspoons Epsom Salts dissolved in about a pint of warm water.

Next day, repeat the dose with one teaspoon of Epsom Salts in another pint of warm water. If you have a bowel motion soon after taking the Epsom Salts, then leave the next dose for a day or two.

Repeat for up to three or four doses taken over a period of four days to a week. This should fix the Candida overgrowth.

You can take two tablespoons once a week to help cleanse the insides and reduce candida.

I find that I do not have to follow such an extreme anti-candida diet if I use castor oil, or epsom salts, on a fairly regular basis.

2) Castor Oil As A Quick Fix For Candida

This works in much the same way as the Epsom Salts cleanse, by removing the effete matter out of the bowel so that there is no old rubbish left around for Candida albicans to breed in. Somehow, Epsom Salts and Castor Oil do not affect the 'good' bacteria in the bowel, which makes them wonderful medicines in treating Candida complaints.

Take 2 tablespoons of castor oil with a cup of black, freshly made coffee, first thing in the morning, before breakfast. You probably won't feel like eating anything much after taking the castor oil. When you do decide to eat breakfast, then eat something light, such as a boiled egg, or a bowl of oatmeal porridge with a grated apple – no sugar, no milk. Fruit is not meant to be good for people with rampant candida. I could not eat any fruit at all for a long time after becoming poisoned with asbestos and heavy metals, but these days I find that eating fruit after taking castor oil or epsom salts works well to detoxify the body of any accumulated toxins and candida. Once you are well, eating fruit should pose no problem.

Wait for a couple of days, then repeat the castor oil dose. This should fix most people's candida overgrowth. However, if your candida is the result of chemical poisoning, then you will have to take the castor oil on a regular basis – once or twice a week, depending on the level of your toxicity. And you will need to be very careful to make sure you avoid all yeasts, sugars, wheat, and dairy products for a time. If you suspect you have chemical poisoning, then seek professional advice from your health practitioner before trying either castor oil or epsom salts.

3) A Third Method Which Is A Quick Fix For Candida: Calcium Ascorbate

Calcium Ascorbate is a non-acidic form of Vitamin C. This treatment works a bit like the Epsom Salts method because it makes the body alkaline. Its effect is almost immediate, like Epsom Salts. Calcium Ascorbate also works to neutralise toxins in the intestines, and to help eliminate those toxins out of the system. These reasons make Calcium Ascorbate a very valuable natural therapy for treating Candida, and for helping to keep the body alkaline and free from disease.

1000 mg once a day with a big glass of water is an appropriate dose for an adult. If the infection is very bad, then you could take up to three doses a day of 1000mg each – just until the bowels start to loosen. Then reduce the dose to between 500mg to 1000mg a day.

4) Using A Warm Water Enema To Help Quickly Eliminate Candida

You can use the enema in conjunction with any other treatment you decide to use. The enema works by washing out the debris from the bowel, so that the candida organism has nothing to feed on. It also eliminates parasites. Walter Last always recommended the use of an enema – daily if necessary – to help cure any disease. I find his advice to be sound. Cleaning the intestines with water does help with candida. Dr. Max Gerson is another healer who insisted on daily enemas to cure his patients of any disease, including cancer.

For the enema, you can add half a small teaspoon of sea salt to around a litre of warm water.

Alternatively, the juice of a lemon can be used in the enema.

Additional Remedies For Treating Candida

Aspirin or White Willow Bark contains salicylate acid: Either of these can be a great help, as can baking soda, if you have a sudden attack of candida which causes pain in the stomach. Both these remedies have an alkaline effect. Two aspirins can be taken with a big glass of water. Or a small teaspoon of baking soda in a glass of water. Use these remedies only as an emergency treatment. It is not good to take aspirin regularly, and nor is it good to use baking soda regularly. Both these things weaken the kidneys, so only use them occasionally.

Calcium ascorbate Vitamin C will also address a sudden attack of candida in the stomach. Interestingly enough, Dr. Gerson used to use aspirin combined with Vitamin C as a pain-reliever for his cancer patients. He found that taking the Vitamin C (which I think was Calcium Ascorbate) helped reduce the toxic effects of aspirin.

Recommended Diet For Candida

The most important thing is not to use reheated food, or to leave food for longer than a few hours in the fridge before using. Freshly prepared food is best.

This is a version of the diet which Walter Last gave to me many years ago.

It is sensible to try to stick to a yeast-free, sugar-free, wheat-free and dairy-free diet. No alcohol, no vinegar, no sauces. Sometimes organic, unpasteurised, fresh milk can be good, especially goat's milk. But generally, it is better to lay off milk and cheese. Soy milk, I find, is often no good because the soy beans have begun fermenting a little in the processing. Beef, fish, chicken and lamb are good. Eggs are good, unless you have a specific allergy to them.

Avoid processed meats such as ham, corned beef, salami and the like. These often have chemicals and gluten in them which can contribute to candida overgrowth.

All green vegetables are good. Raw celery is especially good for candida, as it contains a natural antibiotic-antiseptic and is powerfully alkaline.

Garlic is another good natural antiseptic for candida. Avoid mushrooms – these are a fungus, which is a type of yeast, and all yeasts must be avoided.

Be careful of carrots and other sweet fruits at the beginning of your treatment. The sugar in these can be problematic. But once the infection has been stemmed, grated raw apples and carrots, and cooked carrots, should be okay.

All good oils such as sunflower, olive, grapeseed, and butter are okay. Olive oil is especially good.

Freshly cooked rice is good, but be careful not to leave any leftovers more than a few hours before using. Cooked mung beans I find okay, especially if plenty of garlic and celery are added. Be careful of all sprouted mung beans and other seeds, as they can get yeasts growing on them due to the several days it takes to grow them. If your infection is not too severe, then freshly sprouted and carefully washed mung beans, or alfalfa, should be fine.

Toxic Pesticides, Toxic Herbicides
Household Bleach, Detergents, and other strong chemicals should be avoided. These, like radiation, all affect the balance of yeasts and other organisms in our environment, as well as the human body.
I find that candida problems, which manifest in the stomach and the skin with me, are almost always due to chemical exposure. I am likely to get a bout of indigestion, with stomach cramps, within a few days of people spraying poisonous insecticide about, or herbicides such as RoundUp. An example from my own experience, I have noticed that the local coun-cil's weed killer brings on the candida symptoms.
I believe everybody in the vicinity of the grass-side verges which the council have sprayed will be sus-ceptible to candida infections. Many people will not realise that the cause of their sudden headaches, or flu-like symptoms, or lethargy, or bone aches, or stomach cramps, or bowel disorders, or depression, is directly related to the toxic sprays, such as Round-Up, which have been sprayed at their door. They will trot along to the doctor to get diagnosed with various complaints, possibly even with arthritis which has come on suddenly, and which will be treated with medical drugs to fix the problem. In fact, more drugs are not what is needed in the case of exposure to toxic chemicals and radiation. Avoidance of the pol-luting factor is the long term answer. Megadoses of Vitamin C and homeopathic remedies such as Thuja do much to negate poisons and restore the immune function after exposure to harmful agents.

Chemical sprays or pellets, as well as household fly-spray, bleach, or chlorine cleansers, quickly throw out the balance of bowel flora, which leads to candida becoming rampant. The candida overgrowth, in turn, lowers the immune system even more, after the toxic chemicals have done their work, so that you might be vulnerable to any flu or viruses which happen to be floating about. You will be more susceptible to infection until you have eliminated the toxic chemicals, and combatted the candida so that the bowel flora is restored.

Epsom salts, castor oil, calcium ascorbate vitamin C, and enemas, will all help to remove the chemicals affecting you, as well as clean the intestines of rubbish.

Radioactive Chemicals From The Nuclear Disaster In Fukushima, Japan

These will be affecting people's health on a worldwide scale for many years to come. Radioactive chemicals are very damaging to the body, as we know.

But, it only takes a small change in the air temperature, in humidity, or the level of chemicals in the environment, for candida to become rampant in an environment. The people of Japan and the countries close to Japan, will be affected profoundly, I believe, by this unseen, phantom yeast, because it affects the natural balance of bowel flora, and consequently, affects the immune system.

Which is why, I think, a daily dose of calcium ascorbate vitamin C is a good idea, to allay the effects of radiation chemicals, herbicides and pesticides in the environment. Some things we have no control over, and so we have to do the best we can.

Chapter 21

Ridding The Body Of Electromagnetic Energies

Sensitivity To Electricity And Electromagnetic Energies

Beware of cell phone towers, electricity transformers, and the new 'smart' meters which have high radiation due to microwaves. Limit the use of a cell phones and wireless computers for your health's sake.

There are several very good, sensible remedial measures to take if you have been sensitised to electromagnetic energies, but of course, avoiding exposure to electromagnetic fields is best, if it is at all possible. Sometimes, a change of lifestyle is imperative, especially if you live under high-wires, near an electricity transformer, or a cell-phone transmitting tower. The microwaves which are emitted from new 'smart' electricity meters will damage your health before long if you have to sleep within three metres of the meter box.

It might be necessary to move house if you are being subjected to strong electromagnetic forces from cell phone towers, or high tension power lines, especially if your health is suffering.

Often people ask me why I don't take certain vitamins or 'do something about it', meaning my sensitivity, by using a device which absorbs electromagnetic energies.

Well, that could be useful. However, even though my health has recovered from extreme electricity sensitivity, I take every opportunity to avoid trouble spots when I can.

Any of the following will undermine my health eventually, if I am subjected to their radiation for too long: an electricity transformer, a cell phone tower, or high tension wires, microwave-operated electricity meters, and even cell phones. These things all have the capacity to undermine my health, reduce my immunity to candida and other diseases, and re-sensitise me to electrical energies, even if I was to take the best of remedial measures.

Prevention is always better than cure.

One example of an effect which cannot be lessened by therapies (except by distancing oneself from the source of radiation, or the wearing of a special mask) is the burning to the eye tissues and the nerves, which transformers, cell phone towers, 'smart' electricity meters and power lines all cause.

Remedial measures are all very well, but there is nothing better than avoiding the source of the problem in the first place.

I have often had to make a decision to move away from a house or location when my health has been undermined through things I cannot change.

So, what are the symptoms of electricity sensitivity, or microwave or radiation poisoning? If you find that your nerves are shaky, your bones ache, your hair bristles when near power sources, or travelling in a car, or your hair is falling out, or that you get electric shocks from touching car doors, or metal objects, or even house windows, or you get headaches or your nose bleeds when driving down a road lined with pylons carrying high tension wires, then you have a few symptoms which are most probably electricity-related.

Depression, anxiety, eczema, heart palpitations, and high blood pressure might go along with any of the above symptoms. Cancer, arthritis or Parkinson's disease could develop if microwave or electrical poisoning continues over long periods.

You might like to see a health professional regarding treatment, but some simple steps which I have found to be helpful are the following:

1) Spend as much time as you can 'earthing' yourself. Walking barefoot on grass, especially damp grass after rain or a fall of dew, or walking on damp sand, or paddling in water, particularly sea water, are all very helpful in expelling electrical energies.

Do one of these every day – several times a day if you are severely affected.

2) Walking: Wear soft-soled shoes – leather soles are good, because leather does not inhibit the connection between you and the earth. If the sole is to be a man-made material, then choose a thin soled shoe, as this will 'earth' to the ground better than a thick-soled shoe. Many people suffer needlessly because they spend their days at work, or at home, wearing shoes which do not allow the electricity from the body to naturally flow into the earth. Even if they do get to walk outside on grass or earth, with thick-soled shoes on, the effect is like that of walking on air: they will not receive the health benefits of nature's natural earthing. This results in one experiencing electric shocks from touching things; hair falling out; water retention; or simply in shakes and tremors developing, which is a sign the nervous system is being literally burnt out.

3) Avoid synthetic fibres for all purposes, especially for clothing, bed-linen and bed coverings, carpet and drapes.
Clothing made with synthetic fibres forms an encasement around the body which provides a great conductor for electromagnetic energies. This creates a huge disturbance for the body's own auric body, or energy field: this system is very finely tuned compared to the superimposed one which is created by the wearing of synthetic clothing, and a way of life which prohibits the natural expelling of unwanted energies.
Bed linen and coverings also play havoc with the body's own electrical circuit. These things are bound to cause restless nights, with headaches and anxieties, and nervous twitching of arms and legs, etc.
Even if you do not have a discernable sensitivity to electromagnetic fields, you will find you sleep better

with pure cotton sheets and woollen blankets, rather than their synthetic equivalents.

4) Avoid the colour red, especially for sheets and garments which you will wear for more than several hours at a time. Red or orange equate to the colours of radiation. They excite the body's nervous system and passions. Red sheets most definitely result in unsettled nights, and do nothing for one who wants to sleep peacefully.
Switch to white, blue or green, and avoid the 'hot' colours for the sheets on the bed. The same philosophy, for people suffering radiation problems, should be applied to the clothing which one wears by night and day.

5) On the subject of sleep: It is imperative that you move your bed away from electricity wires which are usually hidden in the wall to provide lighting for you to read at night. This placing of electric wires, right by the head, is the worst place they could be, as they are closest to the brain. Over time, apart from experiencing headaches and migraines, the pituitary and pineal glands could be affected. This can result in hormonal imbalances occurring.
Move the bed to the part of the room which is furthest away from the transformer and trails of electricity wires in the walls. Move the bed out from the wall if you have to, and put your head at the bottom end of the bed if there is no way, in the meantime, to distance yourself sufficiently from the electric currents.
You are better to get a bedside lamp to put beside the bed – this can be turned off at the wall when you have finished reading. Make sure that if you use an extension cord that this is not coiled about you, as this intensifies the magnetic effect.
Overhead lights are usually far enough away from the

head and body to be of concern, however, if you live in an apartment block, you have to consider where the wiring is below you for the apartment beneath. Move your bed away from the main tracks of wires which lead to the lighting of the flat below. The television sets of the neighbours on all sides also needs to be considered. Do not sleep on the other side of a wall where a television is placed, neither in your own flat nor that of your neighbour's.

Avoid sleeping underneath television aerials also – these affect the brain profoundly and, if you are sensitive, will cause memory loss within a short time. I find, when I have moved a sufficient distance away from an aerial, say at least 20 feet, that memory is restored again.

Apartment living, I have found, is particularly disagreeable to my health.

6) Drink plenty of good quality water. This helps in taking away toxins from the body, and also in antidoting radiation – partly in the urination process, which contacts us with earth.

You can solarise your water with the colour green. This helps antidote the red of the radiation which the body has been exposed to. Just fill a green-coloured glass bottle with good water and leave in the sun for five hours. Experiment with different shades of green using different makes of bottles, as the effect of some is definitely better than others, depending on what ingredients have gone into the making of the glass.

7) Bath and shower in fresh or salt water daily – several times a day if needed. Water is the best thing in grounding us to the earth by transporting electrical energies into earth.

Sea water with its salt content is especially healing of electromagnetic troubles.

8) Cleanse the body of toxins as much as you can. Metals and other poisons in the body contribute toward its holding in of electro-magnetic energies. Plenty of fruits and green vegetables are essential.

9) Spirulina and kelp are excellent aids in helping to eliminate radiation sickness. Use also magnesium and calcium-rich foods or supplements. I have found mag.phos., calc.fluor., silica, Vitamin C and Halibut liver oil capsules to be helpful, although I would advise anyone interested to get a professional to advise on the use of these things.
Professional help for the treatment of candida albicans is a good idea: Sensitive people are prone to candida, and also to electro-magnetic vibrations.
However, this should only be a short-term measure, and a long-term solution to the problem of your environment should be sought. Being candida-free certainly makes the body more tolerant to stresses of all sorts, but if you constantly expose yourself to magnetic forces and radiation, the natural beneficial flora in the bowel is destroyed, which means you will be forever buying expensive acidophilus and other things to maintain healthy digestion. I find that avoiding electromagnetic forces is a better way than filling up constantly on the things which have been depleted by radiation.

10) Lying still on green grass whilst doing breathing exercises is a very healing practice.
When my arms and hands were suffering badly, with constant tingling, pins and needles and numbness, I found going out several times at night onto the cool green lawn to touch the damp grass for 5–10 minutes at a time helped the condition enormously.

There have been times in the past when I have been severely affected by electromagnetic energies, but these days I am very sensible about where I live:

I choose my abode as carefully as I can. I am still sensitive to electromagnetic energies and their high-frequency vibrations, but I am not made sick from them, provided I treat them and myself with respect by keeping my distance.

These sensitivities can be put to good use in matters of healing, a subject that will be discussed at another time.

Note: This post was written around ten years ago. Now, there is another issue challenging us all in 2015, and that is the advent of new so-called 'Smart Meters' which have replaced our old analogue systems of electricity meters. The rays from these new meters are affecting my health very badly at the moment. The problem is in having such a small flat where one cannot escape the effects of the microwaves being emitted from these meters: I have not one, but two meter boxes on my lounge wall. It is very much like having two mini cell-phone towers in my living room and kitchen.

It is not so bad having 'smart' meters if you live in a large enough house where you can get at least 7 metres or so away from the meter box. But they are a hazardous thing when your living area is so small that you cannot escape their microwaves. They are very bad for the eyesight, the nervous system, mental health and overall physical health.

One particular New Zealand power company, 'Contact', have been very helpful and removed the microchip from my daughter's meter in Dunedin. Alas, the situation with my house is not so straight-forward, since I do not own the house. Because I have someone else's meter alongside my own one on the wall, I am subjected to an on-going double dose of whatever the authorities have considered to be a 'safe' dose.

Chapter 22

Bee Colony Collapse Disorder And Neonicotinoid Poisons

Bees Killed By Insecticide

This article was first published on merrilyn hope. com on February 6th, 2011. Since then, Holland and Mexico, followed by the European Commision, have banned neonicotinoid poisons. Bayer, who makes and markets neonicotinoid pesticides in Europe, has threatened to sue the European Commission for banning the product and causing loss of sales. Does this remind you of the tobacco scandal? Doctors were pictured on television during the 1950's, smoking like chimneys, telling us they were smoking their favourite brands, and that smoking was good for you because it calmed the nerves. It was many decades before the truth came out.

Isn't it morbidly ironic that neonicotinoid poison is a synthetic form of nicotine which comes from tobacco?

Bees, and other pollinating insects and birds, are essential for life on this planet. Without them, our fruit trees and agricultural crops will not produce any food. All bees are helpful in sustaining life here on Earth: honey bees, bumblebees, solitary bees, mason bees, hoverflies, butterflies, moths, even wasps, and spiders, all play a part in our existence on earth. We should not be killing the insects of the planet.

Information was revealed in a New Zealand Herald article (22/01/11) which points to neonicotinoid insecticides being a contributing factor in the mysterious disappearance of bee colonies around the world. Bee Colony Collapse Disorder reportedly has affected between 20% and 40% of all American hives. The same colony collapse disorder has been noted in other countries around the world, such as France, and Taiwan.

As yet, so the article says, the problem has not hit New Zealand or Britain, though I doubt this very much: We have had our own share of bees falling sick, and hive numbers diminishing, and I think that insecticides must surely be the main part of the problem. But as I wrote in posts around 2010-11, bees, dogs and wild animals such as koalas are also sensitive to electromagnetic radiation, such as that emitted from cell phone towers and cell phones. Italian beekeepers reported on Jamie Oliver's show recently that their bees were being affected by electromagnetic forces. Radar systems, and satellite interference, will be playing a large part in the decline of bees and other pollinating insects.

Bees are also vulnerable to any insecticide, whether it be a neonicotinoid class insecticide, or another type of chemical, or a herbal concoction. Insecticide agents get carried back to the hive by the bee, and this means that all bees in the hive will be affected by the poison. Herbal insecticides should never be used on a plant when it is flowering.
The trouble with the neonicotinoid compounds, imidacloprid, and clothianidin, is that they are systemic poisons. This means that they get into every fibre of the plant, including the pollen. Only microscopic amounts of neonicotinoids are needed for bees to be affected. They carry the pollen home, where it affects the whole of the hive.

Glyphosate weedkiller is also absorbed into the plants wherever it is sprayed.
Microscopic amounts of these pesticides cause bees to become vulnerable to the killer disease nosema. Nosema is one disease which causes beehive collapse. Studies which were done in 2009 showed that bees who had come into contact with the neonicotinoid pesticides had increased risk of succumbing to this disease, and this was even when the insecticide poison could not be detected on the bee, though the scientists knew that the bees had been exposed to it previously.

Neonicotinoid insecticides, which mimic the insect-killing properties of nicotine, affect the central nervous system of the bee, as well as that of all mammals, including humans.

Be forewarned: Nicotine, we know, affects the central nervous system. These synthesised chemicals, which mimic nicotine, will eventually be proven to be affecting human nervous function and our immune systems, as well as those of the bees.

Research which was done two years ago in America, at the American Government's Department of Agriculture's Bee Research Laboratory in Beltsville, Maryland, has only just been made public. The results of this research has been duplicated in another independent study completed by French researchers at the National Institute for Agricultural Research, in Avignon.

A two year wait for this information to be made public surely causes one to wonder as to the reasons why: Many other countries already have bans, or partial bans, on the use of neonicotinoid insecticides, as their use has been linked to the drastic reduction of bee colonies, and other health and environment problems.

The countries which have restrictions on the use of neonicotinoid insecticides are: France, Germany, Italy and Slovenia. But the USA, and Britain, and most likely, New Zealand, Australia, and many other countries around the world, are still using these very toxic insecticides.

Bayer chemicals, which is a German firm, is adamant that its neonicotinoid insecticide compounds are 'safe if used properly'. But there can be no ' safe and proper' use of neonicotinoid insecticides, as incredibly microscopic amounts affect bees and other insects, as studies have proved.

Bayer started making neonicotinoid insecticides around 1990. Some of these neonicotinoid compounds are known as imidacloprid, and clothianidin, which is the latest. Be on the alert for new compound names. No chemical insecticide is 'safe', for either insects or human or animal life.

Bayer reportedly made 510 million pounds, or $1.07 billion, in the year 2009. These astronomical profits will, of course, be an incentive for Bayer, and other companies with their own versions of the insecticide, to continue making and marketing these insecticides for as long as they possibly can.

It looks as if the American government is 'in' on this: a leaked document which came out in November 2011, probably thanks to Wikileaks, showed that the US Environmental Protection Agency had continued to license clothianidin, 'even though its own scientists reported that the tests Bayer carried out to show the compound was safe were invalid', so the New Zealand Herald article says.

This decision on the part of the US Environmental Protection Agency does nothing to protect the environment. Obviously, the big guns are at work here. Money talks, and talk is cheap, apparently: Bayer spokesman for Bayer CropScience UK, Julian Little says 'bees are very, very important to Bayer CropScience and we recognise their importance.' Yet, the welfare of bees is obviously not important enough for Bayer chemicals to discontinue with the production of neonicotinoid pesticides, even when other countries have seen fit to ban them, or restrict their use. Not when they are making them $1.07 billion a year.

Little maintains that neonicotinoid pesticides are 'safe when used properly': He says 'I'm sure there are some very interesting effects Dr. Pettis has seen in a laboratory, but when you get to what's important to everybody [?], which is what happens in the field, you don't see these things happening'.

The main point this Bayer representative overlooks is that bees are affected by such minute amounts of neonicotinoid poison, it cannot be detected by technology as yet. Because the pesticide works undetected, silently and invisibly, it is very easy to ignore and blame the death of hives on other factors.

What Is Being Done In Britain?
The Co-operative Group, which buys farm produce, has banned the use of neonicotinoid pesticides from providing farms. This is an indication that the Co-operative Group recognises the danger to people who consume food which has been treated with imidacloprid or clothianidin.
In January 2011 the Labour MP for Gower, Martin Paton, requested that the government suspend the use of neonicotinoid compounds, following the recent revelations in the US over Bayer's latest neonicotinoid, clothianidin.

'The Strange Disappearance Of The Bees'
This is the title of an excellent film from 2011 by American filmmaker Mark Daniels, in collaboration with Dr. Jeffrey Pettis, who did the research on bees several years earlier at the American government lab, and Dennis van Engelsdorp, who works at Penn State University.

Chapter 23

Boron For Creaky Joints In Cattle And Goats

Natural Remedy For Arthritis, Osteoporosis And Soft Bones: Boron Is Essential For Health

It is a fact that diseases can result from deficiencies of certain minerals and vitamins in the diet.

Disease can result, too, from exposure to herbicides, pesticides, and other harmful chemicals. Agents in these poisons can cause sudden depletion of certain minerals in our bodies, as well as having a harmful, residual effect.

So, let us not use any harmful chemicals, and concentrate on improving the quality of our pastures, animal health, and vegetables by supplementing essential organic elements, so that we all stay healthy. We need only small amounts of certain trace elements, but if these essential trace elements are lacking in our food, then we get sick.

Take a look at how cattle can develop arthritic symptoms, osteoporosis and soft bones when they do not have enough Boron in their diets See how well they recover when given the correct treatment – a boost of Boron to their feed, and some of it applied to the soil.

It stands to reason, then, that the same goes for people – disease can often be cured by taking supplements of the minerals which are lacking in our diets. Pat Coleby's book, entitled 'Healthy Cattle Naturally', which was published in 2002 by Landlinks Press, Collingwood, Vic., Australia, gives valuable insights into mineral and vitamin deficiencies of animals. You can still purchase the book, hopefully, by emailing publishing.sales@csiro.au

This is a very technical book which would be of interest to all farmers and orchardists interested in improving their soil and the health of their animals through natural, organic means.

But for the layman, we can glean so much useful information from this book, as the nutritional science which works for the soil and animals is the same one which works for us.

For many years, Pat has kept a herd of milking-goats which he were kept healthy by adding borax and other minerals to their feed, and seaweed to the soil on which they graze.

In 'Healthy Cattle Naturally', Pat Coleby describes how cattle also become sick when their diets consist of too little Boron. Apparently, around Bendigo, in Victoria, Australia, where the soil has low readings for Boron, all stock suffer arthritis unless the deficiency is addressed.

Because the soil was so deficient in Boron, causing weakness in farm goats' bones and joints, Pat found it necessary to dose the goats with a little Borax each week to correct the deficiency. Page 90 reads, 'I had to add 1 teaspoon a week of Borax per 30 head of goats.' I think this means the dose was 1 teaspoon per goat per week, as a little further on it says that the dairy cattle, although needing less Boron than goats, sometimes needed to have a boost of 'about 5 g (a teaspoon) per head', which was added to the feed just once each week 'with beneficial results'.

Seaweed and Borax, the Sources of Boron

The easiest remedy for a Boron deficiency in the soil is seaweed. Seaweed is rich in Boron, Cobalt, Zinc, Iodine, and Selenium, which are all trace elements necessary for the health of soil, farm animals, plants, and people.

You can see how valuable the daily addition of Boron-rich kelp to our diets will be, for helping to prevent such conditions as arthritis, osteoporosis and other bone troubles.

Borax as a Supplement

The other method of curing a Boron deficiency in animals and soil is to use Borax, sodium borate. Sometimes it is necessary to supplement this as well as seaweed, when the soil is extremely depleted of Boron.

One has to question the quality of the soil on which our supermarket vegetables have been grown. If our vegetables are low in Boron, and other essential trace elements, then, over time, we are likely to develop arthritis and other maladies, just like the cattle and goats around Bendigo.

Pat says that soils which are low in Boron are hard to grow good food on. The ears of wheat do not fill out properly, leaving the lower part of the wheat ear undeveloped. Fruit and nut trees do not thrive. Legumes and lucerne, or alfalfa, will not grow in Boron deficient soil, or soil which is low in Magnesium or Calcium.

Dolomite powder is the remedy for low Magnesium and Calcium.

Pat Coleby's Basic Mineral Lick Recipe

Here is a mineral combination given by Pat Coleby as a general base-lick to keep animals healthy. Pat advises keeping it around for stock to partake of, and also suggests keeping rock salt available for stock to lick. Stock apparently take just the right amount needed of the lick and the salt to keep their health good.

Dolomite 25 kilograms
Copper Sulphate 4 kilograms
Yellow dusting sulphur 4 kilograms
Seaweed meal which is urea free 4 kilograms

Pat insists that the lick must not be allowed to get wet, as the copper content is lost very quickly if it gets rained on.

Chapter 24

Causes Of Memory Loss
And Some Remedies

Too often people say that the cause of memory loss is a genetic thing, especially when it is related to Alzheimer's disease and other types of dementia. But while we accept that some people have a propensity for afflictions of the brain, and memory loss, as with cancer and other degenerative diseases, much can be done, in my experience, to avoid or avert these conditions in most people, even when there is a genetic weakness.

Candida Can Cause Memory Loss

A weakened immune system can result in candida, which can cause memory loss. Toxic chemicals, alcohol, microwaves, toxic dentures, and some medications can cause candida.

It is easy to cure candida: The main thing is to starve it of the foods it thrives on, and avoid all those environmental contaminants which encourage it. Periods of detoxification, as in fasting on raw foods, castor oil occasionally, an alkaline diet, avoidance of all toxic herbicides, pesticides and other substances, and a healthy environment is the way to recover your health and naturally improve your memory.

Heavy metal poisoning, asbestos, addiction to alcohol and other drugs, vaccinations and some medications, as well as agricultural chemicals such as RoundUp's glyphosate, all have the potential to weaken the immune system and incline people to candida infection.

Any of these things, given enough exposure, tend to upset the functioning of the bowel flora, and kill off the very organisms which are there to help digest our food and protect us from sickness.

One incident which caused my own severe memory loss, and a near physical breakdown, was the poisoning which occurred after I cleared a property of asbestos and toxic ash after a fire. I began to suffer from heavy metals, formaldehyde, and asbestos dust poisoning my system. Lead is one heavy metal which is known to severely affect nervous system, brain function and memory, and combined with all the other poisons in this toxic ash, it very nearly caused my death. I guessed that if I wasn't to die of heavy metal poisoning, then I might die of candida.

Candida took over my digestive system to the extent that eating a grain of sugar, or a drop of fruit juice caused an immediate visible reaction in the mouth, which became white with thrush. As long as I did not eat anything which fed the organism, then I was okay. But there was very little food which was safe during this time. Raw lettuce, for instance, was no good, as there are multiple little organisms on lettuce which cause the lettuce to decompose fairly quickly. As my immune system was so incredibly weakened, I had no resistance to the yeasts on lettuce, or the sugars in sweet vegetables such as carrots, or apples, which caused immediate candida overgrowth.

It took a very long while to rid myself of the poisons which were making me ill, and to build up resistance again, but I managed a recovery with castor oil, and a diet which allowed only raw celery and tuna fish in oil, and calcium ascorbate vitamin C. I followed this regime religiously for six months, after which time I was able to eat cooked vegetables again. After this initial healing period, I still had to follow a strict modified diet using both cooked and raw vegetables, tuna fish in oil, and continue to use castor oil for cleansing at least once a week.

Gradually, my memory and physical health was restored.

Childhood Vaccinations

It is probable that vaccinations in childhood play a part in people's immunity being low and too readily succumbing to candida and other infections throughout life. I believe that childhood vaccinations, as well as flu vaccinations, could also be one cause of mental deterioration and memory loss because of their influence on the digestive and immune systems.

Childhood vaccinations could even predispose us to cancer, obesity, alcoholism, and other addictions later on in life. See my website MerrilynHope.com for more information on vaccinations, particularly the article entitled 'Link Between Vacinations and Obesity' from August 2012.

My generation was the recipient of numerous nationwide school vaccinations and innocculations in the 1950s and 1960s. It is no wonder, to me, that so many of my peers have died young of cancer, heart or breathing problems, or addictions, and that many of us still living have suffered from chronic short-term memory loss.

Avoid Exposure To Radiation And Electromagnetic Energies

As stated in the article entitled 'Improve Your Eyesight Naturally', electromagnetic radiation from cell phone towers, 'smart' electricity meters, and electricity transformers, can harm brain function very dramatically.

These vibrations and radiations affect the central nervous system, which runs on its own series of electrical impulses. The nervous system's energy circuit is very sensitive to the stronger rays from things like cell phone towers and electricity meter boxes, and the result of prolonged exposure is that the organs suffer. The brain, eyes, ears and heart, which are all connected to the nervous system, are especially vulnerable to these toxic energies.

These radiations and electromagnetic fields can also cause candida, as they have the ability to kill off the 'good' bacteria in the bowel, to the advantage of the 'bad' bacteria and other parasites.

Anti-Candida Diet Improves General Health And Memory

Important: If you feel at all unwell whilst you try this anti-candida diet, then quit the diet and go back to see your health adviser. However, it can be rather trying at the beginning of the diet, as the candida yeast will demand those sugars and foods which feed it, especially when you are starving it of these items. If you can resist the temptation to eat those foods which candida loves, then after a week or so on the diet, your candida infection should be more or less under control.

The best way to combat candida and rebuild your immune system is to starve it of all sugars for a while. This means adopting a very radical approach which involves more than being gluten free. You need to cut out all wheat flour products – no bread, cake or pastries, as these are all converted to sugar too quickly. Wheat flour, and many other flours, can cause the candida to thrive whilst your immune system is poorly functioning. Cut out sweets, including all sweet drinks, juices, fruit and honey for a time. Dairy products are also best avoided; the lactose in milk, including soy milk, also feeds candida. All leafy greens are just great, as are most vegetables, but cut down on those potatoes and kumara, or sweet potato, and carrots for a while, as these carbohydrates are converted to sugar very quickly in the digestive system, and this gives the candida plenty to thrive on.

Brown rice is generally good; however, if your condition is chronic, then you will need to exclude all grains until you improve. Taking olive oil, rice bran oil or some other good quality cooking oil with your brown rice, and poured over your salads and cooked greens, helps slow down the process of sugar conversion in the body: it is nourishing, and inhibits the candida, because candida doesn't like oils. Taking garlic with your brown rice and oil also helps inhibit candida overgrowth. Use garlic and oil at every meal until you are better. Even after you are better, good oils, garlic, brown rice, salads, and cooked greens should form the bulk of the diet to avoid getting a candida imbalance which causes memory loss.

Protein And Vegetable Oils

A protein-rich diet, and the use of good quality oils such as virgin olive oil, is very effective in combating candida infection. Candida does not thrive in protein-rich diets, and vegetable oils. You must have adequate protein in the diet – candida sufferers are often on vegetarian or low-protein diets where grains are used to substitute real protein. Try to eat protein at every meal. Oily types of fish are the very best – salmon, mullet, sardines, tuna, but free range eggs, almonds, free range chicken and beef, are all good sources. Nuts are sometimes best left until you begin to recover, but you can experiment with these after you have given yourself a week or so without, to see what their effect is. Once you have followed this anti-candida diet for a few days, you can recognise what foods are best to avoid when you try them again, as you usually get symptoms of candida fairly soon after eating them.

Avoid taking protein foods such as soy bean tofu, soy bean miso, and cheese, as these are all fermented foods which encourage candida.

Eat Salad Foods At Every Meal

Celery is very effective in helping to combat candida, as it has plenty of roughage to cleanse the bowel. It is a very alkaline food which makes for a healthy body and immune system. It also has an antiseptic effect which inhibits candida and other bacteria. Celery is a great cleanser and helps to build healthy blood, whilst being excellent for the brain. Sprouts are a great food, but you have to be careful with these as yeast begins to grow on the sprouts while they are germinating: they must be washed well – I think these are best left out until you have recovered somewhat. Lettuce must also be washed well. Avoid tomatoes for a while – they are too sweet. Avocado is best avoided for the first few few weeks until you have strengthened your immune system, as they begin to ferment very quickly and therefore feed the candida if they are overripe.

The other thing which you must starve the candida of is any food or drink which contains YEAST. Candida is a yeast, and it gets a huge boost when you feed it things like alcohol, vinegar, sauces, or even vegetarian products like soy bean miso, tofu, or soy sauce: all these are fermented. Just a taste of another yeast really sets off the candida growing again. Mushrooms need to be avoided, as the yeast on mushrooms encourages candida overgrowth in your intestines.

If you suspect that candida albicans might be the cause of your memory loss, then the above suggestions should be helpful. Remember to eat enough while you are on this diet. There is absolutely no need to go hungry. Have a salad ready, maybe with boiled eggs or fish added to it, and some brown rice, already cooked, which you have put in the fridge. You can snack on these super healthy foods, throw a few almonds in with cooked broccoli or spinach, throw on a bit of olive oil, a taste of garlic, and you are ready to go.

Avoiding all yeast foods and sugars will help your memory loss if candida, or sluggish bowels, is the problem. The bulk of salad foods, cooked greens and brown rice which you eat with your protein will provide good roughage to get your bowels clear of effete matter, get them functioning normally again and provide the very best nutrients to feed your body and your brain.

Using Calcium Ascorbate To Treat Candida
Calcium Ascorbate, or Ester C are the non-acidic Vitamin C types you should look for in treating candida. These are the most effective of all available supplements which counteract candida albicans, and thus they are helpful in restoring your memory. They also help keep an alkaline state in the body which is another important factor in treating candida. Do not use the ordinary, sour-tasting Vitamin C, as this does not help candida, but actually feeds it. Calcium ascorbate in doses of 1000mg can be taken once, or twice, or even three times a day to combat candida and help your memory grow strong. Cut the dose back after a few days, once the bowels have been cleared.

Acidophilus
This is the name of one of the beneficial bacteria in the intestines. Acidophilus helps keep the candida in check, so it is very useful in tackling the cause of your memory loss. Having a healthy amount of acidophilus in your bowel also helps you to process your food more efficiently, thus more nutrients are provided to the brain, helping to counteract memory loss. It is important to find a product which is suitable for candida sufferers, though. Make sure there are no added sugars or lactose added to the acidophilus which you buy. Otherwise it is best to do without.

Epsom Salts For Magnesium
This is very helpful in clearing out the bowel of toxins. The extra magnesium can also boost your brain function. Take a dose several times a week, or as needed.

Bowel Cleanse or Colonic Cleanse
It is a good idea to go to a colonic clinic to get this professionally done at first. After that, you can learn how to use an enema so that you can clean out your

system regularly. This is especially important in the beginning of treatment, when toxins will be released from the liver because of the healthy change of diet you have implemented. Washing out the colon is an important measure to take in getting rid of all the gunk in your bowel: keeping the bowel clean is a priority in helping to build a good memory.

Candida does affect very many people, and most people, given the quantity of processed food which we all consume, have sluggish and clogged bowels. These things are probably the most common causes of memory loss, so the above dietary and cleansing suggestions really are worth a try.

Some Other Causes Of Memory Loss

Emotional exhaustion, lack of sleep, anxiety, and depression: these can all contribute to a state of memory loss. Good nutrition, such as the basic wheatless anti-candida diet outlined above, should help most people with these conditions. Also, Yoga Nidra, deep relaxation and yoga breathing are useful in minimising these negative mental states. See the chapter at the end of the book on how to practice Yoga Nidra.

Radiation from cell phone towers, cell phone use, electrical transformers which are too close to your house, overhead power lines near your house, radio transmitters, even television aerials above your sleeping space, can all affect your memory and your nervous system generally. Having a radio close to your head at night will interfere with your brain patterns and affect your memory: I read once that Paul Simon won't sleep with a radio or a television anywhere near his bedroom, even if it they are not going. He recognises the negative effect radio and television waves have on the brain and memory function.

Alcohol And Marijuana Addiction

The effect of both these drugs is well known to be deleterious to the physical health, and to the mental health. Marijuana has a potent weakening effect on memory.

Allergy To Denture Plastic Or Acrylic

Many people are sensitive to plastic materials: these materials, which are prolific in our environment, are one major cause of memory loss in my experience. Unfortunately, many people wear plastic in their mouths, in the fabric of their denture. This plastic starts to break down after a couple of years or so, and chemicals from the plastic denture are absorbed into the body. This affects the brain and is one of the probable causes of memory loss in people who have dentures. Also, candida yeasts and other bacteria can thrive in the denture plastic, especially when it becomes older, and these bacteria also cause memory loss. See the chapter on Toxic Dentures in this book, for more information.

Essential Vitamins And Minerals

Lack of certain essential elements in the diet such as iron, B vitamins, niacin, pantothenic acid, biotin, Vitamin A, Vitamin D, Vitamin E, Vitamin C, iodine, silica, manganese, selenium to name a few of the important ones. These are all essential to keeping a well functioning memory and a healthy brain.

Chapter 25

Homeopathic Bothrops Can Help Speech After Stroke

Homeopathic Bothrops Lanceolatus

This homeopathic remedy is derived from Martinique's deadly, venomous snake, and is one of the lesser known remedies. It can be used to help stroke victims who suffer speech difficulties such as stammering following a stroke, according to 'Herbal Remedies and Homeopathy', published by Geddes & Grosset, 2001 (see page 204).

I have included it here to give an idea of the amazing scope of homeopathy, and because I thought it could be useful: So many people in my neighbourhood have had strokes recently, or have suffered them in the past. The warfarin they have been taking for years, and which their doctors still prescribe whether or not they have had a stroke, seems to be part of the problem, as I see it. Warfarin is made from the same chemical used in rat poison. It causes haemorrhage in rats and mice, and it possibly does the same thing to people too, after long periods of taking it. Homeopathic Arnica and Vitamin C calcium ascorbate, would surely be a better option as a preventative for stroke, and to help recovery.

Do remember that homeopathic preparations are made quite differently to herbal medicines. The principle of 'like treats like' is the operative phrase in homeopathy. A minute and almost undetectable amount of the original substance is all that is left after the process of diluting and succussing a homeopathic remedy many times.

The Bothrops remedy in homeopathic form is a massively diluted preparation of the venom from the deadly poisonous snake, Bothrops Lanceolatus, which is also known as Yellow Viper or Lachesis Lanceolatus. You would not ever try to make up your own homeopathic remedy from this deadly snake. But the Bothrops remedy can be purchased from reputable makers of homeopathic medicines.

Stroke damage to the left side of the brain:
This causes problems with speech, as well as paralysis and weakness on the right side of the body. These are aspects which occur with people unlucky enough to get bitten by the Bothrops snake. With homeopathy, these maladies can sometimes be reversed or helped by giving the Bothrops homeopathic remedy.

Haemorrhage and Strokes: Homeopathic Bothrops Lanceolatus can also be used to curb the bleeding of haemorrhages of many types. The remedy, therefore, could be useful in preventing bleeding of the brain after a stroke.

Thrombosis: Homeopathic Bothrops is listed in several of the 'Materia Medica' as being a remedy for Thrombosis.

Gangrene: Homeopathic Bothrops is also listed as a remedy for preventing Gangrene after haemorrhage. The venomous bite causes gangrene in its victims, which is why the homeopathic preparation can reverse or help prevent the development of gangrene.

Blindness Caused By Bleeding: Amaurosis, a bleeding into the retina, is one effect of poisoning by the Bothrops venom, so it is very likely that in homeopathic microdoses, the preparation of homeopathic Bothrops could also stem bleeding into the retina.

Other Useful Homeopathic Remedies To Prevent Stroke Or Treat Effects of Stroke Homeopathic Opium: Dr. Caroline Shreve lists Homeopathic Opium if a stroke seems imminent. Opium is a good, basic remedy to have on hand. It can help prevent a stroke. For a slow pulse.

Homeopathic Arnica: Homeopathic Arnica is great for emotional upsets and shocks of any kind. It can be used if you suspect a stroke might occur. Homeopathic Arnica for a fast pulse, difficult breathing and weakness on the left side of the body and limbs. High blood pressure can be an indication of an oncoming stroke. Homeopathic Arnica can help reduce the blood pressure, thus preventing a stroke occurring. If high blood pressure is an ongoing problem, the chapter on the breathing method to reduce blood pressure could be useful.

Baryta Carbonica: Baryta Carbonica can also be used after a stroke, especially with right-sided complaints and paralysis, with tongue and speech affected. Baryta Carbonica has a similar effect to the Bothrops remedy which can help left-side brain damage. Left-side brain damage manifests as right-sided weakness or paralysis, and speech difficulty.

Chapter 26

Calf Liver Broth Provides Enzymes For Cancer Patients

Walter Last put me onto making this enzyme-and-mineral-rich broth for curing extreme debilitation which I experienced after being exposed to the chemical defoliant 2,4,5-T. I also used calf liver broth at a later date, whilst treating a breast lump. The first three weeks of my healing programme were spent detoxifying on juices and raw foods, with porridge the only cooked food (see the details in the programme outlined in Chapter 2 in this book). Then, after about three weeks, I introduced the calf liver broth to rejuvenate, nourish and heal the liver and other organs.

Calf liver broth is an excellent way to nourish the body with vitamin B, iron and other vitamins and minerals which are very expensive to buy as supplements. It is best to take your vitamins via the food you eat: the vitamins in calf liver would be more efficiently assimilated by the body than if you were to take a handful of supplements.

At the present time, I am eating a mainly vegetarian diet, and I don't use calf liver broth. Like many people, I don't like the idea of killing animals for food. However, if you are very ill, then you might temporarily overlook humanitarian principles in order to get well. Basically, you are drawing from the life force of the animal when you use calf liver broth.

Calf liver juice does not sound very appealing, and it goes against the notion that we use all raw foods to get well. However, it is only the juice which is used, which is sipped in teaspoon doses at a time. By not actually eating the meat itself, your intestines are saved from having quantities of meat going through it, which putrefies in the intestines, making more toxins for your body to get rid of. The enzymes in calf liver juice, prepared in the way suggested, aid digestion. A ton of important minerals and vitamins are made easily available to replenish the sick body, and the putrefying aspects of meat are lessened, especially when the calf liver juice is followed by a raw carrot juice or some other raw food.

Recipe For Calf Liver Juice

Take a calf liver and slice it up. Put the pieces into a glass jar which has a screw-top lid, such as an agee jar. Add one cup of water to the liver. Screw down the lid. In a saucepan which is deep enough to hold water to halfway up the jar, place a portion of folded cotton such as an old thin tea towel. Place the agee jar on the cloth and fill the saucepan carefully with water up to the level of the calf liver which is in the jar with its lid screwed down.
Important: Do not forget to put cloth at the bottom of the saucepan, otherwise your glass jar will crack. Put the saucepan over a hot plate on the stove. Turn onto medium. Once the water is simmering, turn down the heat to very low so that you barely see the bubbles coming up in the water. Leave on the stove for about two hours.
When two hours is up, strain the liquid off the liver. Put the liver into a piece of gauze or an old cotton tea towel and squeeze the rest of the juice out. Discard the liver. When the juice is cool, it must then go into another, smaller, screw-top jar and then kept in the fridge.
Sip a teaspoonful or two at least three times a day: ten minutes or so before meals or a juice is a good time, as the enzymes will help you digest your food. Make up enough brew to keep you going for up to three days. Then discard any left over and make a fresh broth.

Chapter 27

Improve Your Eyesight Naturally

The Causes Of Weakened Eyesight

Poor nutrition, inadequate water, environmental toxins, candida, and lack of eye-movement exercise can cause a weakening of the eye-sight. Environmental hazards like formaldehyde, which is found in compacted wood-chip for floors, will cause your eyesight to deteriorate quite rapidly if you are daily exposed to the toxin. If you live in a house which has a particle board floor, then over time, your eyesight will deteriorate, your memory will suffer, and you will probably become depressed with all of this as well.

Petrochemicals, toxic herbicides and pesticides, and isopropanol, used in antifreeze and solvents, are all damaging to the soft tissues of the body, and especially to the eyes. Regular castor oil treatments as used in the Gerson diet for cancer, and higher than normal doses of Vitamin C calcium ascorbate are the best ways to remove these chemicals from the body so that they do no further damage. Epsom salts taken once or twice a week can also be helpful in improving the eyesight, for similar reasons.

Radiation From Cell Phone Towers And Electricity Meters

Electromagnetic rays can ruin your eyes, and in a very short time. If your electricity meter box is situated close to your working space, or on your bedroom wall, then you will be exposed to an intensity of electromagnetic energies which will undermine your eyesight, as well as your memory and brain function. This is a serious problem for people who do not realise the harm they do to their health when they spend long periods at a time being exposed to these rays. The problem has suddenly gotten far worse since the advent of so-called 'smart' meters which are far worse than the old analogue meters. These new meters work on a satellite system which uses microwaves to do the work of the meter-reader. Recently, smart meters have been installed on my lounge wall, and the first reaction I have is burning eyes and blurred vision. This is corrected when I go away for a few hours, out of the range of these harmful radiations.

Even before 'smart' meters, my father-in-law lost his eyesight completely over a three year period, and I believe this was due to sleeping on the wall directly behind where the meter box for their motels was situated. His head was within about a foot of the meter box when he lay in his bed. I warned my relatives about the danger, but they did not believe me. Within three years, my dear father-in-law was totally blind, and they had to sell up their business. Cosmetic eye makeup is generally best avoided if you want to protect your eyesight. If you do use eye pencil, make sure it is a safe product, with no harmful additives. Indian Kohl is safe to use in its pure form.

How To Help Improve Eyesight
Provided you are not constantly being exposed to poisons, then these following ideas will help you to improve your eyesight.

Of course, daily general exercise such as swimming, walking, cycling, or yoga, will help the general health, and your chosen daily exercise will help your eyesight too, because this will get that blood circulating. A healthy flow of blood has the effect of better nourishing the eyes with the fluid, proteins, minerals and vitamins which they need for their healthy functioning.

Exercise also helps to keep the blood clean by working the abdominal muscles: this aids the removal of effete matter from the intestines, so that the blood which reaches your eyes will be free of harmful toxins.

Eye-Movement Exercises

Much improvement in eyesight can be observed (excuse the pun) when such simple exercises as the ones outlined here are done on a daily basis. They really are so dreadfully easy to do, and can take almost no time at all if you practice them whilst travelling on a bus, or whilst watching a bit of television. Don't do them while sitting in your car, though, as you may become so absorbed in your exercises that you fail to see that green light, or worse, the red one.

Many of us city dwellers who have desk jobs, or who pore over books or computers all day long, or mozie around the house once the children have flown the coup, do not use our eye muscles, or the change of focus mechanism, anything like half as much as what we should. Our eyes become lazy, as we get used to working within the same frame of focus for much of the day.

Extreme vertical or horizontal movements of the eyes are made redundant as we fix our gaze on our screens, with something like a short 15 degree angle only being all that is necessary to catch sight of the keyboard, and this at more or less the same distance as the screen from the eyes, which means that the eyes have to do very little re-focussing. Our heads become kind of frozen into a forward-leaning posture when we are thus stuck at a desk or a piano or a television, which does not give us much of a range of distances and angles for the eyes to explore.

Now there is a definite relationship between the movement of the eyes and the nasal and sinus passages: When the eyes become lazy, the nerves and muscles which prompt the sinuses into releasing mucous become lazy too. The result is sinus trouble – a congestion in the nasal area, which directly affects the nerves of the eyes and your vision. Weak eyesight is often the direct result of sinus congestion.

You can test this theory for yourself by doing a few rounds of these yoga breathing eye exercises (see the instructions below). You will notice that the sinus passages will release fluid as you do these exercises. You should keep up the practice for several minutes, with variations, until the sinus passages are cleared of mucous. The muscles and nerves of the eyes will thus be toned up, especially if you practice the exercises on a daily basis, and this will have the effect of strengthening your eyesight.

Circular Motion Of The Eyes: You can do this exercise either sitting or standing. Do not strain the eyes by pushing them too hard initially. Begin by looking straight ahead. You do not move the head for this exercise, but rather make the eyes do all the work. Look up as far as you can to the ceiling. Slowly bring the eyes down in a circular motion, stretching out the angle to the side as far as you can to catch sight of the objects to the side of you. Keep moving the eyes slowly until you are looking downwards as far as you can to the floor. Keep the head erect – let the eyes do the work. Come upwards to the left side slowly, again, reaching out as far as you can with the eye movement so that you see all objects as far to the left as you can. Keep moving slowly upwards. This is one round. Do three rounds, then reverse the direction to do three anti-clockwise movements.

Palm the Eyes: To give the eyes a little rest, rub the palms of the hands vigorously together. Put your warmed hands over the closed eyes for a minute. Breathe evenly and deeply, imagining the vital force from your hands going directly into the eyes to strengthen and heal them.

Vertical Movements: Now slowly look upwards. Stretch upward with the eyes as much as you, can without straining, or course. Breathe in as you reach upwards with the eye movement, breathe out as you slowly draw the eyes down to the floor. Breathe in as you raise the eyes to the ceiling. Do three rounds.

Horizontal Movements: Moving the eyes slowly, again whilst keeping the head still, look to the far right. Bring the eyes back to the center and then slowly move the gaze to the far left, trying to focus on something each time. Come back to the center. Repeat three times. Coordinating the breathing with the exercise gives more power to the exercise. Breathe in as you look to the side, and out as you return the gaze to the center.

Head Rolls: This exercise stimulates the blood flow to the brain and to the eyes. It also helps the flow of chi down the spine. Simply drop the head forward onto the chest. Breathing in slowly, slowly move the head towards the right shoulder. Keep moving slowly upwards, rolling the head gently backwards, over the top of the spine, and over to the left shoulder. Your lungs should be full of air now. Slowly begin dropping the head down from the left shoulder as you breathe out. Keep moving down until the head touches the chest. Repeat three times, then reverse the direction.

Head Drops: Now, breathing out, drop the head sideways onto the right shoulder. Breathing in, lift the head back up to the erect position. Do three times. Drop to the chest as you breathe out, lift up as you breathe in. Repeat three times. Drop the head the same way to the left shoulder, slowly, three times. Drop the head backwards as far as is comfortable. Bring to the erect position and repeat slowly twice more.

Diagonals: Next, look up to the very top right corner of your field of vision. Bring the focus downwards to the centre so that you are looking straight ahead. Keep moving the eyes in a diagonal direction until they are looking down at the left hand corner. Come back slowly to the centre and continue up towards the top right hand corner. Repeat until you have done three rounds. Repeat the whole exercise beginning at the top left hand corner. It is, again, more beneficial if you can coordinate the breathing with these exercises. Breathe in as you look up, and breathe out as you draw the eyes to the floor. Keep the breathing fluid and steady, with fluid and steady eye movements accompanying the breathing.

Acupuncture

Acupuncture given to relieve sinus congestion will very often have the effect of sharpening your focus and improving short and long-focussed vision. Visit a registered acupuncturist to get advice on this. Alternatively, you could do self-acupressure to help the situation: Massaging the points on and around the eyebrows, at the side of the eyes, and the point directly under the eyes, below the pupil, can help relieve sinus congestion and stimulate the blood to the eyes.

Improve The Bowel Function With Epsom Salts

Taking a dose of Epsom salts once or twice a week keeps the digestive tract clean and removes toxins from the bowel and liver. A deficiency in Magnesium can affect the eyes, and this is easily corrected with regular doses of Epsom salts which contain Magnesium.

Lutein is another nutrient which is especially good for the eyes. My neighbour was recently prescribed lutein by her eye specialist, which she gave my friend for macular degeneration. What a breakthrough, to have this nutrient recognised by the medical profession. It can be found in leafy greens such as spinach and kale, but is also present in lentils, peas, beans and tomatoes.

Extra Vitamin C in the form of Calcium Ascorbate is also beneficial for the eyes. This improves digestive function, removes acidity from the body, and helps to neutralise and remove toxins from the body.

Iodine: Dab a couple of drops of Iodine on the skin or scalp once or twice a week. Iodine is also important to keep good eyesight.
Eat enough good quality protein and plenty of green vegetables and fresh fruit.

Carrots are one of the best vegetables for the eyes. They contain lots of Vitamin A which is essential for healthy eyes. Carrots were fed in megadoses to World War I and II pilots to increase the efficacy of their vision.

How Cancer Of The Retina Was Reversed Through Diet And Improving Lifestyle
This is an excerpt from my website article published May 23rd, 2012
http://merrilynhope.com/vitamin-c-megadoses-for-cancer-as-alternative-to-surgery-radiation-and-chemo/
'My sister who is a naturopath just told me this morning that her friend was diagnosed with cancer of the retina a few months ago. She came up to Auckland hospital to see a specialist who told her

she would have to have her eye out. This advice really freaked her out and had the effect of her changing her attitude and devoting herself completely to a health regime to reduce the cancer, using every natural means possible. After several months of her changing her lifestyle, getting onto a healing diet, detoxification, and even giving up her job for the meantime while she restored her health, she has had confirmation that the retina cancer has reduced by around half already.'

Here are some additional details on how this person reversed her eye cancer:
Along with raw foods, a little fish was used, plus feta cheese and raw egg yolk. No meat was taken.
Prayer and vital force exercises, such as pranayama breathing, were practiced.
Milk thistle, the maximum allowable dose, was taken daily.
Other herbs and supplements included:
Dandelion and globe artichoke.
Gentian gymnema.
Digestive enzymes for the pancreas.
Selenium.
For the immune system: Cat's claw, Astragalus worsania, Rodeola, Poke root.
After two months, this person went back to the specialist who had wanted to remove her eye. He could not believe that the cancer had shrunk from 5.2 to 3.6 mm in that time, simply by following 'natural' cleansing methods, combined with a nutritionally rich, organic diet.
No conventional pharmaceutical drugs or preparations were used, and the end result of her 'natural' healing effort meant that she did not need surgery.

Chapter 28

Iodine Scalp And Hair Remedy

Iodine Tonic For The Health Of The Hair

Iodine is a wonderful, natural, relatively inexpensive item for restoring hair growth and improving the scalp tissue.

As well as the iodine treatment, a good nutritious diet should be followed. Taking castor oil orally once a week can help with hair growth. Have plenty of good protein foods, such as oily fish, free range eggs, plenty of fresh green vegetables, and make sure your food contains enough B Vitamins. The calf liver broth for cancer, which I have given the recipe for in this book (see Chapter 27), would be a good way to up your B vitamins, niacin, and iron. If you apply iodine on a regular basis to the head, you not only nourish the scalp but the whole body as well, as iodine is absorbed gradually through the tissues of the scalp and into the body where it is utilised to help immune function, the improving of which helps to stave off diseases like cancer and arthritis and makes minimal the effects of flu, colds and other infections.

Generally speaking, if you are healthy, then you should have a good head of hair. Generally speaking, if your hair is thinning or falling out rapidly due to sickness, shock, or old age, then you should look first to iodine to help restore the hair and the general health simultaneously.

In the 1950's, when I was growing up, iodine was commonly used by our mothers so that we would not become iodine deficient and become sick. Our mum would paint the soles of our feet once a week or two, or we would get dosed with iodine via a cut on a hand or leg, where my mother would douse the iodine.

At some stage, common salt became iodised so that we would get enough iodine in our diets. If you do not use salt, then I would say that you are possibly iodine deficient, in which case the Iodine Scalp-Hair Remedy will be an ideal way for you to take extra iodine into your body and nourish your hair and scalp at the same time.

If you continue to use this Iodine scalp treatment, then you should expect to see favourable results after several months, when new hair should be starting to grow. I myself have found the iodine scalp treatment to be very effective.

Of course, you can overdose on iodine – sensitive people or those who have low blood pressure or who exercise too little need less iodine on the skin in order to absorb what is necessary for hair maintenance and healthy immune function. People who exercise a great deal, or swim regularly, can take more iodine on the skin, as much of what is applied will be sweated off in exercise or in the water.

The best thing is to use moderation in using Iodine as a scalp-hair remedy: too little is better than too much. Too much iodine absorbed through the skin can give you heart palpitations, hot flushes and anxiety if you are at all sensitive to chemicals. However, remember that iodine is a necessary component for good health, so do use it, but use it carefully.

Method for Using Iodine as a Scalp-Hair Remedy

After washing the hair, you can apply a little iodine. Just three or four dabs of the finger to the bottle is enough. Each time you dab, put the iodine on a fresh part of the scalp. Then, once you have applied your three or four dabs to the area you are treating, massage with the fingertips all over the scalp. With the massage, you actually transfer small amounts of iodine to the whole head of hair. Massage serves to increase circulation to the hair follicles, which also helps hair growth, and stimulates the kidneys and other organs simultaneously.

Always use the Iodine scalp-hair applications after washing the hair, as if you wash the hair soon after-

wards, much of the iodine will be washed away. Try
to leave the iodine on the hair without washing it
for a couple of days or so to give the iodine a chance
to be absorbed into the scalp and into the body.
Two or three dabs of Iodine could be applied to the
scalp twice a week, no matter what your body size
or condition. After the next wash, dab the iodine to
another part of the scalp. In this way, you ensure
that all parts of the scalp eventually get treated.
Note: Eucalyptus oil and Apple Cider Vinegar are
also good to encourage hair growth and nourish
the scalp, but do not use these on the same days as
you use the Iodine on the hair. The reason you do
not combine these treatments is that if either one
of these items is mixed with iodine, unpleasant and
slightly toxic fumes are emitted which can have
the effect of making you dizzy. Then you will feel
compelled to rush off and wash everything, iodine,
eucalyptus, cider vinegar, the lot, which would ren-
der your treatment useless.
If you use cider vinegar after washing your hair to
neutralise the alkaline effect of soap or shampoo,
then wait until the following day before you apply
any iodine, or at least 8 hours, I would say.
The Iodine scalp-hair remedy is also very effective
in keeping head lice and other lurgies at bay. There
again – if the hair and scalp are healthy, then head
lice are not likely to be drawn to it.
Iodine has the effect of acting as an insecticide
as well as helping to improve the general state of
health of body and hair. The other important thing
in treating head lice, though, is to use apple cider
vinegar after using soap or shampoo on the hair.
Head lice love scalps which are alkaline, either from
using alkaline products like soap or shampoo, or
from using too many acid-forming foods in the diet.
If your child or yourself have succumbed to head
lice, then DO use apple cider vinegar after each
wash. In this case, you will apply the iodine to the

scalp the following day or 8 hours later.

POSTSCRIPT: I recently received a query via my website: 'I have spilt either iodine or hair dye on my white floor. How do I get this terrible stain out?' My advice is: Hair dye causes hair to fall out, which is why you would not use it if you are seriously trying to improve hair growth. Toxic hair dye damages the liver and can lead to cancer: Jacqui Davison found she had a build up of hair dye in her liver, which was expelled with castor oil when she began a serious fasting programme to rid herself of cancer.
About that stain: Try baking soda, slightly dampened with a lot of elbow grease.
For your hair: powdered henna is a natural, non-toxic dye and should be okay.

Chapter 29

Gall Bladder Cleanse With Apples, Olive Oil, And Lemon Juice

Natural Remedy For Treating And Preventing Gallstones Or Constipation

Here is a very effective and easy-to-do method for preventing gallstones. It will expel existing small gallstones and help to break up larger stones. Do it just once in a while to keep the gallbladder free of stones and stale bile.

It is also useful as a detox which will help to remove toxic chemicals from the digestive system. This makes it a helpful treatment for chronic cases of candida, especially when exposure to toxic chemicals has occurred.

Of course, do see your doctor or naturopath if you are experiencing any pain to do with the gallbladder.

The raw apple, olive oil and lemon treatment is also effective for stubborn cases of constipation. Because of its great detox effect, it is a good thing to do occasionally for prevention of bowel cancer and other maladies caused by auto-intoxication, such as arthritis.

Walter Last recommends a similar method for expelling gallstones, and I have tried it myself with good results.

So – one of the best methods for a gallbladder flush is outlined below.

Raw Apple, Olive Oil and Lemon Juice Gallbladder Cleanse

Three Days On Apples: Begin the treatment with eating only raw, grated apples for three days. Raw apple, grated with its skin still on, cores and all, has a wonderful healing effect on the digestive system. It is roughage-packed, full of Vitamin C and other antioxidants, as well as phytochemicals which help prevent cancer.

You can eat some whole apples as well with the diet,

but grate them also, so that you eat plenty as a salad at mealtimes.

Each night while you do the raw apple days, take one tablespoonful of olive oil with some lemon juice – and a spoonful of lecithin if you have it.

Don't worry if you don't have lecithin, as the oil and lemon will work as a cleanser, even without it.

On the third apple day, take 1/2 cup of olive oil with 1/2 cup of lemon juice, mixed together. Swallow the lot down in one dose. It is surprisingly easy to take when lemon juice is combined with the olive oil.

There is an option of using orange juice instead of the lemon, but lemon juice is more acidic, more antiseptic, and is a quicker-acting remedy.

Straight after you have swallowed your olive oil and lemon drink, lie on the right side for two hours with a pillow under the hips.

The Castor Oil Pack: The other thing you can do on the days you are eating only raw apple is to use Castor Oil on a pack. You put this on the outside of your stomach/gall bladder area. The pack is easy to make. First buy a bottle of castor oil. Pour around 2 tablespoons over a white cotton or woollen cloth – not too big, just big enough to cover a good area of the stomach.

You leave the Castor Oil Pack on overnight with a piece of plastic over it, and something around the outside, like tightish pants, to hold it there. You can loosely bandage it in place if you want to.

Every night, on the nights you take your raw apple, put the Castor Oil Pack on the stomach. Leave it on for the whole night.

Save the castor oil pack each morning to use again the following night. Put a little more oil on occasionally to keep it moist.

You do three nights on, and take it off during the day. Even after you have taken the Olive Oil and

Lemon to eliminate stones, you can keep up the routine with the Castor Oil Pack to ensure the healing of the gallbladder.

The same routine pattern applies after you have finished the raw apple and olive oil treatment: Three nights in a row with no pack, then three nights on again with the pack.

You can use the Castor Oil Pack indefinitely in this way – three nights on, three nights off. No pack during the day-time.

Good Foods to Aid Gallbladder Function and Prevent Gallstones

Drink plenty of water each day; less coffee and tea, and more water.

Eat fewer animal fats and products. Eat more of the healthy Omega-3 fatty acids which are contained in oils such as olive oil, fish oils, and linseed or flax oil. One to two tablespoons of any one of these oils per day is a good preventative measure against developing gallstones.

Try to incorporate olive oil as a daily commodity in the diet.

Eat plenty of fibre-rich foods, such as fruits, green vegetables, beans, lentils, nuts and seeds. More fibre in the diet will take away the unwanted cholesterol from the system. Since gallstones are apparently made up of, mainly, cholesterol, more fibre is essential to prevent stones from forming.

Apples and pears are especially good for the gallbladder, as well as for improving bowel function.

Try to avoid wheat products, such as breads and cakes. Avoid pasteurised dairy milk and switch to either raw milk, if it suits your digestion, or soya milk.

Chapter 30

Two Week Cleansing Detox Herbal Recipe

Natural Herbal Remedy And Cleansing Tonic

Simple to make and simple to use; here is a two-week cleansing formula to help start the new season with more vitality.

This is a silica-rich herbal tonic which uses comfrey, dandelion, birch leaves, nettles and rose hips. These herbs, in combination, can improve the digestive system as well as improve the hair.

This herbal remedy works as a cleanser by encouraging the elimination of harmful toxins from the liver and intestines. It can also be effective in helping to reduce fat deposits.

This formula can help constipation. It can help to purify the blood. It can also help reduce the pain of arthritic and rheumatoid conditions.

This herbal tonic will also help to improve the digestion by removing mucous from the bowel and toning up the liver, so that nutrients from food can be absorbed more easily.

The herbs used in this recipe are rich in iron, potassium, silica, enzymes, vitamins, serotonin and other nutrients which will help build good blood and nourish the body cells, bones, hair and nails. Nettles and comfrey are famous for their silica content which builds strong bones, helps encourage hair growth, and to form strong healthy nails.

Recipe For Herbal Cleansing Tonic

Mix together equal quantities of dried birch leaves, comfrey leaves, dandelion leaves, nettle leaves and dried rosehips. Use around 2 tablespoons of each dried herb. Mix, and store in an air-tight container.

To Use The Herbal Cleansing Tonic

Take one rounded teaspoon of the herbal mixture and pour over a cup of boiling water. Let the tea infuse for 10 minutes before drinking.
Take the tea twice a day for two weeks only.
Cease taking the cleansing tea after two weeks.
Wait for at least a month before you use the two-week herbal cleanse again.

Enema Or Colonic Cleansing

It is helpful, though not imperative, to take an enema or two during this period of cleansing. Washing out the bowel of toxic residues lessens the chance of getting headaches or other unpleasant symptoms which sometimes arise when toxins are released through fasting and cleansing.

What To Eat Whilst On The Two-Week Herbal Detox

Breakfast: Have a large bowl of oatmeal porridge in the mornings with a grated apple and olive oil or a little butter.
Lunch or Dinner: Eat plenty of cooked and raw greens, rice or potatoes, and good quality protein in the dinner meal, such as free-range chicken, free-range eggs, and fish.
Healthy Snacks: Snack on fruit, nuts, seeds, and soya milk, if these are tolerated. Almonds, sunflower seeds and ground sesame seed are very nutritious, rich in calcium and iron, and make good snacks or accompaniments to salads and healthy desserts.

Foods To Avoid During Cleanse

If you can, for best results, avoid wheat bread, cakes, sugar and dairy milk whilst you are on your two-week herbal detox.

Chapter 31

Suspected Lip Cancer Healed With Vitamin C, Garlic, Homeopathic Ledum and Dairy Free Diet

Alternative Treatment For Basal Cell Carcinoma

This alternative remedy for a type of skin cancer took some time to work, and much concentrated effort. This is how I recently healed a lip cancer using a detoxification diet, enemas, and megadoses of Vitamin C, Garlic Oil and Homeopathic Ledum.

My lip developed a major hole around October last year (2013). A lot of RoundUp herbicide, which contains glyphosate, was being sprayed around the flats where I lived, and about the town on all the grass verges. Spraying seemed to occur every two to three weeks. This stuff always affects my health adversely.

This was also a time, the beginning of spring, when I was doing a lot of gardening, and using commercial potting mix and so-called organic fertiliser. The hole just would not go away, no matter how I kept it out of the sun, and no matter what sort of healing balms I applied.

I did notice that each time I went near the bags of organic fertiliser, and the plants I had bought, which had commercial potting mix in them, my lip became inflamed and sore. I could feel the lip tingling in objection to my gardening materials. It was also worse each time glyphosate was applied onto the grass near my flat, and worse for any exposure to the sun.

So, I gave away all the organic fertiliser I had on hand, and moved my pots well away from the house. That helped for a start. I always wore a sunhat and even a scarf, to protect the lip from the sun's rays. If I had to go shopping, I took an umbrella. This strategy went on for months, while I took several trips to the doctor to get a diagnosis and where I was given several prescriptions for creams which had no good effect at all.

I was lined up to get a biopsy done at the hospital, which proved to be a very interesting, if not bewildering experience.

An appointment was finally made, a year later, after I had finally healed the lip through natural treatments. I decided to go along and have them look at the lip which was scarred, and some lesions on my back and legs. A biopsy was done on a back lesion. I went back a few weeks later and was told that the test results showed basal cell carcinomas on the back and legs. I wondered about their diagnosis, because they did not biopsy any part of the legs. The specialist said that the lesion on the lip would have been basal cell carcinoma too, but that it had healed spontaneously, as they sometimes do.

Of course, it was not a 'spontaneous' healing: I had worked very hard, applying garlic and ledum throughout the day, taking massive doses of Vitamin C, avoiding wheat and dairy, and using internal cleansing methods.

They gave me a prescription for a chemotherapy cream which I was told I must use if I wanted the lesions to heal. I suggested that if one lesion had healed 'spontaneously', the one on my lip, then perhaps the other ones might heal too, with the same natural treatment I had applied. No, the chemotherapy cream is what you need, they said, but be careful with it.

I did not take the prescription into the chemist, but decided to follow my own therapy again, and eliminate milk and wheat, to heal the other spots on my legs, arms and back. These eczema areas had become better while I was practicing my healing methods, but once the lip was healed, I had relaxing my efforts, allowing milk and wheat back into the diet, and so the other areas had worsened again. These so called carcinomas, according to the local doctor I saw in the beginning of my quest for help, have appeared on areas which have had excessive exposure to sun over the years, with the result that the skin is damaged.

The most perplexing part of this story is that two weeks after the last visit to the hospital specialist, when I was given the chemotherapy prescription, I received a letter from this specialist. The letter said that I 'must not use the chemotherapy cream on the back, because that was not basal cell carcinoma', but that I must 'use the cream on the legs, because that was definitely basal cell carcinoma'. But I was never tested for basal carcinoma on the legs, so how could they assume this? They were obviously just guessing. I decided they had no idea what they were talking about, and that the only way I was to get better was through my own efforts.

How I Cured Basal Cell Carcinoma On The Lip

Vitamin C: Between 6000 mg and 10,000 mg of non-acidic Vitamin C were taken each day. I used whatever deals were cheapest – calcium ascorbate tablets of 1000mg and ester C powder. I took a tablet or two every two or three hours through the day. This dosage was kept up for three to four weeks. Then, on seeing how the carcinoma hole was getting smaller, with scar tissue showing on the edges, I reduced the dosage slowly to around half the original dose.
Then, around another month on, I reduced the dose to just a couple of 1000mg tablets per day, taken morning and night. The Vitamin C treatment took around three months.

Garlic Oil: This proved to be very effective, taken internally and also applied topically over the sore lip. I bit a capsule open every few hours and applied the oil over the sore, then swallowed what was left of the capsule. I carried on applying garlic oil to the lip for around three months.

Homeopathic Ledum Cream: Around twice or
thrice a day, in between the garlic oil applications,
I applied homeopathic Ledum cream. This had a
wonderful soothing and healing effect. Right away
you could feel the coolness of the Ledum, and the
therapeutic effect it was having on the skin.
I continued the Ledum treatment for around three
months, by which time the lip was healed.

Castor Oil: I took castor oil around once a week,
to clear away toxins from the liver and intestines.
Castor oil also has a healing effect on all parts of the
body, as it seeps through to all body cells and helps
to distribute nutrients. So that – combined with the
neutralising effect on toxins, and its cleansing effect
– makes it a remarkable healing agent.

Cut Out Wheat Milk and Sugar: These were
all eliminated from my diet whilst I was healing my
lip. Instead, plenty of greens, soy milk, good quality
protein and oatmeal porridge with grated raw apple
formed the basis of my diet. I allowed myself one
good cup of brewed coffee per day, but took great
care not to get the hot cup near my lip. Heat on the
lip was the worst thing, I found, so I reduced my
hot drinks and used a straw to drink my coffee.

Homeopathic Thuja And Arsen Alb: I used
both these remedies for periods, using one remedy
at a time. Mainly, I used homeopathic Arsen alb.,
as this remedy seems to work well for me as an
immune-booster. Whenever I feel a dose of flu or
a cold coming on, I take Arsen alb. right away, and
the flu is either avoided completely, or abated.
After a week or so on Arsen alb., taking a few drops
two or three times a day, I would switch to Thuja
instead, and take that for a few days. Thuja has a
remarkable effect on the body by helping to neutralise poisons such as RoundUp and other herbicides

and insecticides. It is also good for the side-effects of vaccination.

Grated Raw Apple: As well as the grated raw apple, eaten with a bowl of oatmeal porridge each morning, I ate one or two raw apples, grated before lunch and dinner. Occasionally, I missed out on the lunchtime apple, but I always made sure I had raw apple at dinner-time. Altogether, I ate around four to six raw apples per day.

Dr. Max Gerson used raw apple with oatmeal porridge in his famous cancer treatment. He also used castor oil as part of his treatment, two tablespoons taken every second morning, followed by a cup of black coffee. I reduced the castor oil dosage this time, for the lip carcinoma, although I have strictly followed Gerson's castor oil method in the past, for healing a breast lump.

Chapter 32

How Enemas Can Help Cancer And Arthritis

Cleansing The Liver And Intestines With An Enema To Aid Healing

Most people abhor the idea of using an enema. Even in a life-or-death situation, touch and go, they just cannot bring themselves to putting water up the bowel.

I have known many people who have died from cancer who, although they made some effort to-wards a 'natural' cure by eating more salads and drinking freshly prepared vegetable juices, would not face up to what was the real problem – toxins in the liver and bowels.

It has been said by many a healer that 'all disease originates from the bowels'. This I believe to be a true enough statement. The best way to keep good health, provided that you have enough food and that you are not exposing yourself to harmful chemicals, is to look after the bowels and keep them working properly.

What most people do not realise is that when you begin to detoxify the body by introducing more raw vegetable salads and juices into the diet, that the rapid release of toxins from the liver begins. When these harmful chemicals begin to leave the liver and other organs, they flood the bowel. So it is impor-tant to clear these chemicals and effete matter as quickly as possible. Otherwise, as these poisons travel through the digestive system, they get reab-sorbed again, through the walls of the intestines and into the blood. And then back to the liver again, eventually.

When this release of harmful toxins occurs, once you begin your cleansing diet, you may suffer symptoms of auto-intoxication and suffer a further decline in health unless you use an enema to quickly clear away those poisons.

Years ago I had a valuable lesson in the necessity of enema use from my healer friend Walter Last.
I had become very ill after 2,4,5-T aerial spraying. My young son who was with me at the time also suffered with chronic eczema and digestive problems. Then, just three months after she was born, my baby daughter died of mysterious sickness, thought to be cystic fibrosis, but never established as a fact. She had the same breathing difficulties which I had suffered from since the spraying, which was similar to asthma.

After she died, feeling my life force severely reduced and ebbing by the day, I went to see Walter Last in Whangarei.
Walter put me onto a great diet which was around 90% raw, with no wheat or dairy products at all except for butter. He also instructed me to use an enema daily.

I decided that I would follow everything he told me to do. Except for the enema. I just would not tell him that I had no intention of using an enema.
For the first couple of weeks, I made an amazing recovery. It was so exciting. I felt I was going to live after all. But then, suddenly, I began to get the most awful stomach pains and felt extremely ill again.

Back I went to Walter.
Well, I did not need to explain anything at all to him. He knew just from one look at me as I went into his clinic, that I had not used an enema.
He angrily shouted at me as he grabbed an enema from his shelf for me to purchase, thrusting it into my hands:

'If you don't use this, you needn't bother coming back to me'.

Nothing more.

I felt incredibly ashamed that I had ignored his expert advice and had attempted to deceive him. I left the clinic right away, after paying his secretary for the enema and the visit.

The use of the enema had a remarkable effect on my health. To this day, especially during those times when I have suffered ill-health such as that which came from asbestos and heavy metal poisoning, or exposure to RoundUp's glyphosate, or other life-threatening health issues, I have used the enema with great benefit to my health.

The enema is especially beneficial for people who accumulate mucous in the bowel, such as celiacs, and others who have allergies to wheat or dairy foods, or who are especially sensitive to toxic herbicides, insecticides and pesticides.

The enema is especially good for treating cancer, arthritis and other degenerative disease, for the reasons mentioned above.

Dr. Max Gerson, who treated thousands of patients successfully with his alternative cancer treatment, maintained that the enema was essential in their recovery. After some experimentation, he would not treat a person without the use of an enema.

Dr. Gerson found, before he began the use of enemas in his cancer treatments, that many of his patients began to get well on the special dietary regime he set out for them, but that, just as I had experienced, became very ill two weeks or so later after beginning the treatment. The initial improvement stopped, and his patients would suddenly give up the ghost and die.

He realised that the poisons being eliminated by the liver were responsible for poisoning his patients, as the poisons were being reabsorbed as they travelled through the bowels. So he introduced the enema

treatment.
After establishing the cause of sudden death in his patients, and so beginning regular enema treatment along with his dietary regime, he found most of his patients improved greatly; and his success rate in treating cancer with his natural means grew enormously.

Chapter 33

Castor Oil And Ginger For Weight Loss

Ayurvedic Treatment For Weight Loss

Here is an interesting but rather nauseous recipe for reducing weight. It uses castor oil and ginger tea and is recommended for people who are 40lbs or more overweight.

Note: NOT recommended for young women who wish to emulate the half-starved look of a magazine model. This recipe is meant for people who have serious weight issues.

I discovered this new use of castor oil in 'Prakruti – Your Ayurvedic Constitution', a book by Dr. Robert E. Svoboda, published by Geocom Limited, Albuquerque, New Mexico, 1989. See page 97.

The method of Max Gerson's, which uses castor oil every second day, is familiar to me for treating serious degenerative illnesses such as cancer. I believe that Dr. Gerson's castor oil method would also work for obesity.

But the method of Dr. Svoboda's described below might work even more quickly to get rid of any unwanted fat.

Method For Using Castor Oil And Ginger Tea

Dr. Svoboda's recipe uses a tablespoon of castor oil each morning, taken on arising. This is continued for six weeks. The castor oil is swallowed down at once with a cup of strong ginger tea which is made from powdered ginger.

Apparently, castor oil and ginger tea taken this way does not encourage looseness of the bowels. But it will start to eat away the fat layers, which is what we want if we are more than 40 lbs overweight.

I think that taking castor oil and ginger each morning would have an effect on the appetite, making you less hungry. This quenching of the appetite might be one of the key ways in which the castor oil and ginger tea method works.

Exercise: Remember to exercise properly whilst you are on a weight loss programme. You need at least 30 minutes of solid exercise several times a week, and preferably each day.

Water, Tea, And Coffee: Fluids should be cut down so that you drink only when you are thirsty. Coffee should be cut down, or cut out if you can, since it is dehydrating. Coffee drinking has the effect of producing protective fat around the gut, in order to protect the liver which becomes dehydrated with too much coffee drinking. I know from experience that this is so.
You do not need to carry a water bottle with you everywhere like the athletes do.
Dr. Svoboda recommends reducing water intake whilst on your weight loss programme (but do check with your doctor before reducing your water intake).

Eat Nourishing Foods In Moderation: Do not starve yourself to lose weight. Crash diets are not the answer, and neither is cutting out fats. We need fats to stay healthy, because fats are needed to process other foods and vitamins. Try and eat balanced meals with good quality protein, green vegetables, and small portions of root vegetables.
Eat plenty of sprouted grains.
All cooked grains can be used in moderation except for wheat. This should be cut out completely. Switch to rice and cornmeal in place of wheat. Wheat is one of the main causes of obesity, as well as many other health problems. Walter Last maintained in the 1970's that New Zealanders were sick principally because of their diet which consisted of too much wheat, sugar, bread, milk and cheese.

Read the following article on the benefits of soy for reducing weight:
http://merrilynhope.com/soya-for-weight-loss-and-lowering-cholesterol/

Avoid Chilled Foods: Ice cream should be avoided, as should all other cold foods. This is because the body regards cold foods as a reason to put on weight, in an effort to preserve heat. It will act defensively to counteract the cold foods and drinks by increasing fat layers. Dr. Svoboda thinks that cool air-conditioned rooms should be avoided for the same reason.

Hot Is Good: Anything which heats the body up is beneficial for losing weight: saunas, jogging or other exercise which makes you sweat, and the 'hot' spices such as ginger, turmeric, chilli pepper, curry dishes, and warm herb teas.
All these things – exercise, the hot spices, the herb teas – heat the body up whilst increasing blood circulation, which is helpful in losing weight.

Avoid Oversleeping: Dr. Svoboda believes that sleeping to excess is one of the chief causes of obesity in people. He suggests slowly, over several weeks, reducing the amount of hours spent sleeping to not more than six per night. He also says that one should never have naps in the daytime whilst you are trying to lose weight.
Some therapists believe that lack of sleep is a major cause of obesity. Be sensible, I say. Get enough sleep, but don't lie in unnecessarily.
If you cannot sleep at night, then you should get up and do something, or read for half an hour. But you should avoid eating anything, or making a cuppa. Keep your fast going through the night, until you take that castor oil swallowed down with your cup of ginger tea in the morning.

Try and go to bed at the same time each night, and arise at the same time each morning, preferably around 6 AM.

More uses for castor oil are outlined in the following article:

http://merrilynhope.com/ideas-for-using-castor-oil-2/ This post was published in May, 2015.

Also, see this older post which I retitled 'Castor Oil Laxative':

http://merrilynhope.com/ideas-for-using-castor-oil/

Apples And Cider Vinegar As A Natural Remedy For Losing Weight

Apples, and Apple Cider Vinegar, are age-old remedies which have been commonly used to help normalise weight, regulate the bowels, strengthen the heart and overall, to improve the health.

The Apple Diet is a great cleansing technique to follow for a few days. Eating only raw, grated apples for three days can help to reduce the weight considerably.

Apples are a wonderful food. They are an extremely nourishing, healthful food which helps the health in a myriad of ways.

However, while eating an apple a day keeps the doctor away, using vinegar made with apples may not suit all people

It is not recommended that people suffering long-standing candida use apple cider vinegar. They should stick to eating fresh apples, if fruit sugar is tolerated, and most certainly should avoid fermented foods of any kind, including apple cider vinegar. See the section below for an explanation on how yeast allergies can occur.

What Are The Healthful Effects Of Eating Apples, Or Using Apple Cider Vinegar?

Apple cider vinegar, which is made from the whole

apple, skin, pips and all, contains all of the valuable nutrients inherent in the apple, but you have to remember that it is a fermented food which may not suit everybody.

Apples, or cider vinegar, have the ability to neutralise an acid body and restore the pH level to normal. They are useful in preventing hypertension and they can help to lower high blood pressure.

Apples have the ability to lower blood cholesterol.

Apples, and Apple Cider Vinegar, are rich in potassium, phytochemicals and other agents which strengthen the immune system and help prevent cancer.

Apples are good for the heart.

The pips of the apple contain laetrile, also called amygdalin, or Vitamin B17, which is used in some natural programmes to treat cancer and other degenerative disease. You can eat a few pips each day to help prevent such diseases. Eating some apple pips each day could also be helpful in reducing weight.

For the average healthy person who does not suffer candida problems, cider vinegar does not have any harmful side effects, as do some other methods for reducing weight. Normal people of a robust constitution can safely use a daily dose of apple cider vinegar for weight control without any fear of adverse reactions.

Cider Vinegar As A Daily Tonic And Remedy To Reduce Fat

It is best to take your apple cider vinegar for weight loss first thing in the morning, before breakfast or coffee. Take two tablespoons in a glass of hot water. Apple cider vinegar, taken each morning, will help to expel any parasites living in the intestines or elsewhere.

It is an acidity regulator which helps to balance the acid-alkaline ratio of the body, known as the pH

level.
It helps to neutralise harmful toxins in the vital
organs and blood. The liver, gallbladder, pancreas,
kidneys and intestines all benefit from the antiseptic and nourishing effects of apple cider vinegar,
taken on a regular basis.
Cider vinegar is beneficial for all parts of the body:
It helps strengthen the bones and nerves. It helps
eyesight. It strengthens the brain and it can help
prevent and improve alzheimer's disease.
It is wonderful for the hair. Taking apple cider
vinegar daily, and rinsing the hair with it after each
wash, helps encourage hair growth.
Applying it to the hair while wet after washing gives
the hair a lovely sheen and helps to prevent head
lice from settling in.

When Not To Use Apple Cider Vinegar Or Vinegar Of Any Kind

Some people are extremely sensitive to yeasts of
all kinds, and their systems are not suited to take
vinegars of any kind.
An extreme sensitivity and aversion to yeasts can
arise if a person has suffered major damage due to
toxic chemicals, such as heavy metal poisoning, or
asbestos poisoning, or poisoning from formaldehyde, asbestos, heavy metals, or agricultural chemicals.
This is not a common problem, but if you have been
exposed to large amounts of these toxins, or perhaps herbicides and pesticides, chronic candida can
strike, in which case you might need to avoid even
apple cider vinegar for a while.
Candida feeds on yeasts of all kinds, including those
which are used in the making of vinegar. So, in the
case of chemical poisoning, when candida overgrowth is chronic, it may be that you have to wait
to detoxify somewhat before cider vinegar can be
tolerated. Some people may never tolerate it.

Chapter 34

Why Do Dogs Get Cancer?

It is not an uncommon thing these days for animals to get cancer. Household pets who are well cared for, still often succumb to cancer. Herbicides, pesticides, and the current trend to vaccinate household pets, all contribute to increasing the incidence of cancer in dogs and cats. Vaccinations in humans have been linked to autism, alzheimer's, depression, arthritis, obesity, cancer and other degenerative conditions, so it follows our pets will also become more vulnerable to these diseases after vaccination.

But even animals in the wild are now suffering higher rates of disease. Soon after I first published the gist of this article on my website, Channel 3 TVNZ featured a nature programme which showed a koala being treated for cancer in Queensland, Australia. The vets on the programme said that they often treated koalas for cancer. This was around 25th September, 2010.

Agricultural chemicals and industrial pollution surely must be the reason that koalas, living in the bush of Queensland, are getting cancer. Glyphosates which are found in the common weedkiller RoundUp have been linked to cancer. WHO have said that glyphosate 'probably' causes cancer. (see reference in Chapter One) This herbicide is used widely in New Zealand, in and around parkland areas, and probably the same goes for Australia too. It is quite probable that a few cell-phone towers and other transmitting devices are located in the vicinity of the koala bushlands. These emit harmful radiations which can cause cancer. Global warming and the erosion of the ozone layer might be a factor too.

There is almost always a catalyst, a toxic chemical which can be identified as the cause of cancer. If it isn't toxic chemicals in the air and on the land, it could very well be some poisonous product we are using or putting on our bodies. Jacqui Davison, who famously recovered from terminal cancer and regrew her hair and teeth in the process, had her cancer analysed. Results showed that her cancer had developed from her toe nail. She had kept her nails permanently painted with nail polish, which is loaded with formaldehyde, one known cause of cancer.

Well, nail polish won't be the reason for cancer in those koalas, or our household pets, but there are some obvious ways in which dogs and cats can get poisoned. Here are the main ones:

Vaccinations.

Herbicide such as RoundUp, sprayed onto grass verges where dogs and cats may walk.

Chemicals in food, such as agricultural herbicides, growth hormones, and antibiotics in animal feed which is given to chickens, sheep and cows. Preservatives, artificial flavourings and flavour enhancers in dog and cat food are also bad.

A diet high in processed food which is deficient in important life-giving minerals and vitamins.

Toxic flea killers and de-wormers. The poisonous flea collar is one of the worst culprits. The poor animal has to continually absorb the chemicals from such, all the day and night long.

Most insecticides which are used to de-flea cats and dogs are incredibly toxic. Harmful chemicals should never be used anywhere in our environment, but toxic flea collars and potions have an added hazard. You have to remember that every time you pat your pet you get some of the poison from its coat or flea collar on your hands. These flea killers are made to be absorbed readily through the dog's skin, and they are just as readily absorbed through your own skin too.

A seemingly harmless thing such as a flea killer will have ongoing negative effects on you and your pet which cannot really be measured. The harmful effects of a simple little flea killer are big. Cancer and arthritis, multiple sclerosis, parkinson's disease, are some of the serious degenerative diseases which can be caused from chemicals found in many poisonous flea killers.

It might take several years for sickness to develop in your dog, or yourself, because of a poisonous insecticide which you use regularly on your pet. But it is inevitable that your pet will eventually suffer with the use of harmful pesticides on his or her skin.

Toxic Pesticides Can Cause Depression
Pesticide use also affects the emotional and physical states of your pet. Your pet is affected immediately upon coming into contact with flea poisons. Poisonous flea collars and powders usually have the effect of making your pet feel ill. Have you noticed your dog getting depressed, losing her appetite, looking sad and moping around, or getting hyperactive after applying flea-killing chemicals to its coat, or giving it a pill, or putting on a flea collar for the eradication of fleas?

You see the same effect on cats and dogs, who often get jittery after having flea killers put on them. You often see them in a frenzy, trying to rub this stuff off on the grass immediately after they have had an application of poison, or a flea collar put on them.

The two main long term effects of using toxic chemicals on your pets, or giving them poisons internally, are arthritis and cancer. Types of muscular dystrophy are also not uncommon in dogs and cats. Depression, hyperactivity and diseases of the nervous system can also develop when toxic chemicals are used regularly on your pets.

The answer is 'no' to poisonous chemicals. We must stop using harmful chemicals on our pets, or anywhere in our environment.

There are organic products which will do the job of getting rid of fleas. There are home-made remedies

which we can make to kill fleas or to deter them.
These remedies may not be quite as effective as the
harmful commercial poisons, but it is far better to
have the odd flea about than risk getting cancer
or arthritis yourself, or have your dog or cat suffer
these diseases.

Poisoning From Unknown Herbicides
The legal spraying of poisonous herbicides such as
glyphosate around parks and pathways is a serious
problem. While people are still allowed to use toxic
chemicals wherever they choose, we have no control over our own exposure, or the exposure of our
children and pets to these toxic chemicals.
But dogs and cats are especially at risk, because,
since they do not wear shoes, they absorb the chemicals which are sprayed on the grass straight into
their paws. Herbicide use around parks and grass
verges in the city poses a real threat to all dogs and
cats living in the area.
On farms, dogs are at risk when paddocks are
sprayed with chemicals, as are the animals who will
eventually get to eat the grass. All toxic herbicides
and insecticides should be banned. Only natural
organic, or herbal, or homeopathic herbicides and
pesticides should be allowed, especially where food
is produced, or in the cities where people, and dogs
and cats roam. That means there is no suitable or
safe place for the use of any toxic chemicals.

Chapter 35

Breathing Method To Help Lower Blood Pressure And Relieve Stress

The Yoga Cooling Breath – Sheetali Pranayama

This is a yoga technique to enhance vitality, induce mental calmness and normalise blood pressure. Sheetali Pranayama is an age-old practice which is included in the teachings of Satyananda.

Sheetali Pranayama will noticeably reduce high blood pressure even after one or two practices of the method. Over time, if you practice it regularly on a daily basis, you will find that your general health will improve, and that your blood pressure will also improve. Of course, attention to the diet and minimising any activities which cause your blood pressure to rise are also important in achieving a balanced state.

Basically, this is a very easy exercise to perform. There are some added sophisticated yoga techniques which you could add to the exercise if you wish to take your yoga practice seriously.

But here I will give the simple, basic method which is effective in calming the mind and in helping to reduce blood pressure, and which anyone can do easily without any prior knowledge of yoga technique.

First, make yourself comfortable, either in a chair, or in your favourite meditation pose.

Take two or three slow deep breaths to clear your lungs of air and prepare for the Sheetali Pranayama cooling breath.

How To Perform The Sheetali Pranayama Cooling Breath

So now you are seated comfortably. Stick out the tongue a little, and make it into a tube shape. You are going to breathe in through this tube made by the folds of the tongue. Note: This is the only one of Swami Satyananda's yoga breathing techniques whereby the breath is taken inward through the mouth, and outward through the nose. It is the

reverse of the usual method.
So, with the eyes closed, we take the breath in
through the curl of the tongue, slowly and evenly.
Hold the breath in briefly with the mouth closed.
Then exhale evenly out through the nose.
Repeat.

Be Cautious – Build Up Slowly

In the beginning, if your blood pressure is high, it
might be best to perform only about three or four
breaths using this curled tongue technique. Otherwise if you do too many at once, you might feel
awfully light-headed or dizzy as the sudden burst of
oxygen into the bloodstream takes effect.
As your strength improves with building up your
Prana, or nervous energy, you should be able to
perform more breaths in the one sitting. In conjunction with regular pranayama practice, nine
rounds is suggested by Swami Satyananda.
For people suffering high blood pressure, Swami
Satyananda recommends building up the practice
slowly for anything up to sixty rounds.

Many Benefits

I find that the Sheetali Pranayama Cooling Breath
has many benefits. As well as the obvious effects
in calming the mind and normalising the blood
pressure, it also oxygenates the blood, helps the
eyesight, enhances the intuitive faculties, improves
memory, and helps to improve the digestion. You
will notice right away that saliva secretions increase
as you perform the exercise. Stimulating the salivary glands in this way greatly helps the digestion.
After a few days of practicing the Cooling Breath,
you will become aware of other more subtle changes which occur throughout the system.
It can be a helpful technique for people suffering all
kinds of degenerative disease, such as cancer and
arthritis.

Remember To Drink Plenty Of Water Daily
This helps keep the blood pressure stable. Take
a glass of water immediately after performing the
Sheetali Pranayama cooling breath exercise.

Jalandhara Bandha – The Chin Lock
If you wish, you could perform the Jalandhara
Bandha as you practice the Sheetali Pranayama
Cooling Breath.
You need to sit in a meditation pose for this, knees
touching the floor if possible, and with the arms
straightened out, hands holding the knees. Hunch
up the shoulders so that the arms can become perfectly straight.
Close the eyes. You then inhale through the curled
tongue, then, close the mouth whilst holding in the
breath, and push the head forward so that the chin
touches the chest.
Hold this position, with the breath retained inward,
for as long as is comfortable. Then, still retaining
the breath inside, slowly relax the pose, bringing
the head up. Exhale slowly through the nose as you
sit with the head erect.
Repeat.
It is important to remember that the head must
be properly erect before breathing in or out. No
breathing should be done whilst the head is down
on the chest in the chin lock.
Personally, I think that the chin lock is a bit much
for most people who are not used to yoga practice,
and who simply want to improve their blood pressure. In my experience, this breathing exercise
achieves results, even without doing the chin lock.

Zip Up The Chakras

After doing Pranayama, or any exercise for enhancing the vital force, you can try this simple one
minute exercise which helps to retain energy and
balance the chakras. It can also be done on its own
to relieve stress at any time of the day and to improve concentration.

Sit comfortably. Close the eyes. As you breathe
in, take the forefinger and middle fingers together,
and slowly but firmly trace a line up from the top
of the pubic bone, moving upwards towards the
chest. Continue on up until you reach the lower lip.
Breathe out. Repeat three times on the inhalation.

Chapter 36

Yoga Nidra For Deep Relaxation And Calming Emotions

Yoga Nidra: A Technique For Deep Relaxation

Yoga Nidra is a deep relaxation technique which the yoga teacher Satyananda has promoted widely in his teachings. It is extremely effective and is very easy to learn. The more you practice it, the better your breathing will become and the more oxygen your body will take in. It releases tensions in both body and mind through the directing of the awareness in a disciplined way.

You will achieve peace of mind through the regular practice of Yoga Nidra.

It is effective in changing patterns of behaviour when it is practiced regularly and can therefore be useful for those who wish to stop smoking. It helps to halt the negative thought patterns of our minds. Yoga Nidra is a very beneficial exercise, not only for those who are giving up smoking, but for all who want to improve health and stabilise thoughts and emotions.

It is an exercise which can inspire and influence people around us because of the good it promotes within ourselves. Our aura becomes more vibrant and clear with Yoga Nidra, and this energised auric body touches the people we meet and affects everything we do. The practice of Yoga Nidra can help shape events in our lives which will benefit others as well as ourselves.

The following is my own adaptation of Yoga Nidra as taught by Swami Satyananda. If you want, you can omit the visualisation section, but I have found this to be most helpful especially when people are sick, lonely or grieving.

This exercise is done with the eyes closed, but you can do it with these instructions in front of you until you become familiar with it. Even this should be helpful.

All you need is half an hour in a quiet space where you can remain undisturbed. Lie on the floor. You

can cover the body with a light blanket.
This is 'savasana', or 'dead man's pose'. Put the
arms alongside the body, slightly away from the
trunk and thighs so that they do not touch the body.
The palms are facing upward and the forefinger and
thumb lightly touching. Legs are on the floor with
the feet slightly apart from each other, not touching.
Close the eyes. Begin breathing slowly and evenly.
Count the breaths and say 'OM' to yourself as
you breathe out. This must be silently spoken to
yourself, as chanting or speaking while in a prone
position is hurtful to the larynx. Chanting exercises
should always be done in an upright position.
Watch the tummy rising and falling with each
breath. 'One' as you breathe in, 'OM' as you breath
out. Feel your body relax totally as you breathe
out. With each breath, the body is becoming more
relaxed. Continue up to TEN.
Keep the even, regulated, deep breaths going. The
tummy rising and falling.
Now, we are going to move through the body with
our awareness. Don't worry if you feel you can't 'get'
it or that you are out of touch with the parts of the
body which we name. It doesn't matter. You just
carry on with the routine anyway and move onto
the next body part.
Take your awareness to the right hand thumb-
----forefinger-----middle finger-----fourth
finger-----little finger-----palm-----back of the
hand-----forearm------outer lower arm-----upper
arm-----shoulder-----right arm pit-----right side of
the chest-----right side of the stomach-----right hip-
----right thigh----knee-----shin-----calf muscle-----
ankle-----top of the foot-----sole of the foot-----right
big toe-----2nd toe-----3rd toe-----4th toe-----5th
toe-----the whole of the right foot lying on the floor.
Keep the even breathing going. The tummy rising

and falling. Feel the body becoming more relaxed on the floor.

Bring the attention to the left hand thumb-----forefinger-----middle finger-----4th finger----- little finger-----palm-----back of the hand-----wrist-----forearm-----outer lower arm----upper left arm-----shoulder-----left side of the chest-----left side of the stomach-----left hip----left thigh-----left knee-----shin-----calf muscle-----ankle-----top of the foot----sole of the foot-----left big toe-----2nd toe------3rd toe------4th toe-----5th toe-----the left foot lying on the floor.

Be mindful of the breath. The tummy rising and falling as you keep breathing slowly and deeply. Totally relaxed.

Come back to the awareness of the feet on the floor. Bring the awareness up the backs of the legs, slowly as you continue your breathing, to the thighs, the bottom, the lower spine, on slowly up the spine until you reach the neck. Keep breathing deeply and slowly. Bring the awareness up the back of the head to the top of the skull, the forehead, the temples, the eyebrows, eyes, cheeks, nose, mouth, lips. Remember to keep a relaxed smile on the lips.

Repeat the whole exercise from the beginning – three times to this point. Now hold the awareness in the eyebrow centre. Watch this space for anything you might visualise here. Now leave the eyebrow centre. Move the awareness slowly around the body in a wide circle. Take your time. Just listen for sounds in the direction you have your awareness placed. No need to analyse these sounds. Simply hear, be aware, and move on your radar sensor further round. Listen for the sounds again. Keep this practice up for a few minutes.

Be aware of the breathing again. Nice, slow, even, energy filled breaths. Watch the tummy rising and falling with each breath.

Now visualise the moon coming up over the water.

You are feeling totally at peace with yourself and
the world. Watch the moon for a minute or two, rising up over the water.
Now you are walking through the garden of Paradise. Birds are singing. You can hear a stream
nearby as you walk down a winding path which has
all the plants in the world growing alongside and
round about it. You can smell the beautiful fra-
grances from many different flowers As you walk
along the path of the garden of Paradise, you can
see a rock pool where a little waterfall is running
gently down. You sit here for a moment and breathe
in beautiful, cool, moist and fragrant air which
heals and soothes you with each breath.
Higher up the path, you can see a Cathedral and
hear Angelic voices singing. All the people you love,
departed and living, are here, making their way
with rejoicing up to the Cathedral. You can decide
whether or not you want to continue further up to
greet them.
Leave your friends and come back to the awareness
of the body on the floor. Hear the birds outside.
Move the awareness around radar-like again, but
more quickly this time.
Move the awareness now to the throat. Keep
breathing. Feel the throat relaxed. Move to the
chest. Keep breathing. As you breathe, feel the
chest relaxed and toxins and negative thoughts and
feelings leaving the body. Come to the stomach.
Breathe. Again, feel negative emotion leaving the
body, and energy from your breath infusing the
area. Move on down-----the hips-----the thighs----
-the knees-----shins-----calf muscles-----ankles---
--tops of the feet-----soles of the feet-----both feet
lying on the floor.
Be aware of the legs on the floor, the trunk on the
floor, the head on the floor. Continue to breathe.
The whole face is totally relaxed. You are smiling
contentedly. Bring the awareness to the eyebrow

centre. Feel at peace within this centre. Keep breathing evenly as you think of the thing which you would like to improve in yourself or within the world. Say a prayer for friends, family and the people in the world who have a need greater than our own. Pray, then, that we might get help with the changes we wish to make in our lives.

We might ask that all patterns of addictive behaviour will cease and that our waking moments be filled with creative, constructive, loving thoughts and actions which will benefit not just ourselves, but those around us.

Say your prayer three times. Give thanks for the blessings in our lives three times.

Prepare now to finish the yoga nidra practice. You can speed up the process of identification of body parts. Take the awareness to the whole body on the floor, the head on the floor, the arms, the trunk, the legs, the feet on the floor. Bring the awareness up the back of the legs, calves, thighs, bottom, spine, head, back of the head, top of the head. Face, neck, arms, chest, stomach, hips, thighs, knees, shins, calves, ankles, tops of the feet, soles of the feet, ten toes. Do this section three times.

Move the hands on the floor. Stretch the fingers. Move the head side to side. Move the arms, wriggle the toes, move the feet. Feel the whole body lying on the floor. You are leaving the yoga nidra state now.

Sit up with your eyes closed. Say 'OM' aloud three times. Chant the sound in a relaxed, long breath. Your tone will be clear and strengthened by the yoga nidra practice. Open your eyes.

Thankyou. Yoga nidra is complete.

Chapter 37

How Art Can Cut Violence In Schools And Harmonise Society

The visual arts, architecture, music and dance, all have the capacity to enhance the life and change the world. In this chapter we look at the example of one school where creativity in the form of an art programme helped to change the school's dynamics for the better, as well as learning outcomes.
Making art, as well as seeing it, has a profoundly beneficial influence on a child's development. I have always believed this, and so I encouraged my children to paint and draw pictures from an early age. Needless to say, they have all proven the truth of this statement. The value of encouraging children to express their emotions and thoughts through art is of great importance in developing the spiritual, higher nature of the individual, as well as enhancing the creative and intellectual aspects.
High art and architecture can help produce a more harmonious society:
Art and architecture, gardens and music, all have the capacity to draw out the best in us. Our surroundings are very important, and we would all do well to improve and beautify our immediate environments as much as possible.

The social value of art and architecture has been recognised since ancient times. Vitruvius, who lived from 70–80BC to 15AD, wrote the only surviving major literature we have on classical architecture. This is a ten-volume treatise entitled 'De Architectura'. He insisted that civic architecture must be solid, useful, and beautiful. His ideas were, much later on, taken up by the Early Renaissance artists and architects: Leon Battista Alberti (1404–1472), who redefined and published his own version of Vitruvius' 'Ten Books' in 1452, and Leonardo da Vinci (1452–1519), and Michelangelo (1475–1564) all held a common belief that High art and architecture contributed to the moulding of a harmonious society.

The 19th century architect and designer, A.W.N.
Pugin (1812–1852), wrote 'Contrasts' in 1836.
Pugin, who has had an enormous influence on civic
and church architecture, both in England, Ireland
and the colonies, 'redefined architecture as a moral
force, imbued with political and religious meaning.'
(See Rosemary Hill, God's Architect: Pugin and the
Building of Romantic Britain, published by Penguin.)
Pugin is another architect who firmly believed that
'good' architecture and design were conducive to
Higher thought and aspirations.
Rudolf Steiner, the early 20th century Austrian psychic and educator, believed that bringing emphasis
to the creative aspects of a child's learning will
result in a more balanced, thoughtful, and caring
child. Art, music, and dance, he said, developed the
soul of the individual.
Steiner schools have a great emphasis on art, with
children using colour, first with crayons, then later
on with paint, as part of their daily routine. Steiner
schools do not teach the intellectual side of education until the child is seven years old. They do not
have formal lessons in reading before that time, but
are read to instead. The idea is that you must not
force the intellect in learning 'stuff' until that intellect is developed fully enough to easily assimilate
and process information.
Until the age of seven, the education is entirely
made up of making things, making art, singing,
dancing, being read to, and learning through play.
By promoting the creative process through art, music and play, the spiritual qualities in the child are
given nourishment, and this encourages harmony
within, so that by the age of seven, they are ready
for the more academic pursuits in education.
To simplify his philosophy, children brought up in
an artistic environment such as Steiner proposed,
are more likely to develop into happy, well-rounded

individuals who will have an interest in shaping a more harmonious society as adults.

There are Steiner Schools in many countries today. Though not a Steiner School, the recent example of Orchard Gardens School in America proves that negative social behaviour can be transformed through art, that learning outcomes can be advanced through art programmes, and that happier children are the result. See the BBC News Report 'Power of Art: Can painting improve your grades?' from the 26th March, 2013, which tells of the social transformation which took place after Andrew Bott's radical new art programme was implemented in his school.

Orchard Gardens is a Boston public school for children aged from kindergarten to year 8. The school is situated in Roxbury, Massachusetts, USA. It has been a violent and troubled school for many years, with a very low academic achievement overall.

Many of the children are disadvantaged economically and socially, and come from a disparate mix of cultures: 56% Hispanic, 42% Black, and 2% Asian. These young children have been in the habit of carrying weapons to school, and so security guards were employed at the school in an effort to check violence and other antisocial behaviour.

New Art Programme For Orchard Gardens Pilot School: In 2010, Andrew Bott became the new principal to the Orchard Gardens Pilot School. Upon his appointment as principal, Andrew Bott immediately fired the security guards. He believed that the watchful security policemen were not improving matters, and were contributing to an environment of mistrust, suspicion and violence.

Getting rid of the security guards removed a lot of tension and created a happier space for the children. But the underlying problems of underachievement and unruly behaviour had to be addressed.

Andrew Bott had a vision of creating harmony by inspiring the pupils through art. Using the money saved from paying security guards, he began to establish an extensive art programme for the school. This new art programme, in just three years, has helped to turn around the outcomes. Peace now reigns at Orchard Gardens School, and the children are much happier. Academic achievement has risen dramatically. Students who were once 'wasters' with no hope for the future, now do their best to keep out of trouble and expend their energy on achieving good and useful things.

The headmaster, Andrew Bott, walked us through, in the BBC interview, onto the third level of the school building, pointing out that although there were 900 pupils studying in the classrooms right at that moment, all was perfectly quiet.

The children now look forward to life, to going to school, and their expectations for their futures have grown.

Art has dramatically changed their lives.

Note: As well as implementing this great art programme to encourage a feeling of self-worth through creativity, which also helps learning outcomes, the learning hours were also extended to improve the academic level.

If we are to raise caring, intelligent, happy, constructive children, we should ensure they spend a good proportion of their learning time in making art, music, and things of beauty. They also need to be read to on a daily basis.

As well, children should have frequent visits to well-planted parks, and civic buildings such as art galleries, and be involved in the planting of gardens.

Connecting with nature, making art or music, and enjoying beautiful art and architecture are all helpful in soothing the soul and aiding the development of the spiritual and creative qualities within us.

Time out to reflect, enjoy nature, and create art of

some kind, is very important for everybody who desires health and happiness in life.

Thus, with more emphasis on artistic pursuits in our schools, more art, music and dance at home, with less time on computers, television and smartphones, we could, in time, achieve a more harmonious and caring society.

Bibliography

Anon. Herbal Remedies and Homeopathy, Geddes & Grosset, New Lanark, Scotland, 2001.

Choudhury, Dr. Harimohan, Indications of Miasm, B. Jain Publishers Pvt. Ltd., New Delhi, reprint 1999.

Clark, Dr. H.R., The Cure For All Cancers, New Century Press, California, 1993.

Clarke, Dr. J.H., The Prescriber: How To Practise Homeopathy, B. Jain Publishers, Pvt. Ltd., New Delhi, reprint 1991.

Daniels, Mark, The Strange Disappearance Of The Bees, 58 minutes, colour, distributed by Icarus Films, New York, 2011.

Davison, Jacqui, Cancer Winner: How I Purged Myself of Melanoma, Pacific Press, Pierce City, 1977.

Dewey, W.A., Practical Homeopathic Therapeutics, B. Jain Publishers, Pvt. Ltd., New Delhi, reprint 1996.

Farrington, Dr. H., Homeopathy And Homeopathic Prescribing, B. Jain Publishers Pvt. Ltd., New Delhi, 1986.

Finkel, M., Fresh Hope In Cancer, Health Science Press, Bradford, England, 1978.

Gerson, Dr. M., A Cancer Therapy: Results of Fifty Cases, Totality Books, California, 1958.

Heinerman, Dr. J., Miracle Healing Herbs, Prentice

Hall, Sydney, Australia, 1998.

Hill, Dr. E., Why Be Scared Of Cancer, G.W. Moore Ltd, Auckland, New Zealand, 1979.

Holford, Dr. P., Burne, J., Food Is Better Medicine Than Drugs, Piatkus Books, London, 2006.

Jeffreys, T., Your Health At Risk, Axiom Publishing, Stepney, South Australia, 2005.

Last, W., Heal Yourself: A Practical Self-Help Manual of Natural Healing, Penguin Books, Australia, 1984.

Levy, Dr. T.E., Curing The Incurable: Vitamin C, Infectious Diseases, and Toxins, LivOnBooks, Henderson, USA, 2002.

Mae, E., Loeffler, C., How I Conquered Cancer Naturally, Harvest House Publishers, California, 1975.

Ministry of Health, 'Task Force on Chronic Agricultural Chemical Poisoning Notifications: Report to the Director-General of Health', June 1986.

Satyananda, S., Asana, Pranayama, Mudra, Bandha, The Bihar School Of Yoga, Monghyr, India, 1969, 1983.

Svoboda, Dr. Robert E., Prakruti: Your Ayurvedic Constitution, Geocom Limited, New Mexico, 1989.

Tenney, L., Today's Herbal Health, Woodlands Books, Brisbane, Australia, 1983.

Vogel, Dr. H.C.A., The Nature Doctor, Bookman Press, Melbourne, 1956, 1995.

Wagner, Dr. E.M. with Goldberg, S., How To Stay Out Of The Doctor's Office, National Library Of Australia, 1994.

Weston, P., Cancer: Cause and Cure: A 20th Century Perspective, Bookbin Publishing, Adelaide, South Australia, 2000, 2003.